BE BRIEF. BE BRIGHT. BE GONE.

BE BRIEF. BE BRIGHT. BE GONE.

CAREER ESSENTIALS FOR PHARMACEUTICAL REPRESENTATIVES

David Currier
with Jay Frost

Writers Club Press
New York Lincoln Shanghai

Be Brief. Be Bright. Be Gone.
Career Essentials for Pharmaceutical Representatives

Writers Club Press
an imprint of iUniverse, Inc.

For information address:
iUniverse
2021 Pine Lake Road, Suite 100
Lincoln, NE 68512
www.iuniverse.com

ISBN: 0-595-17418-3

Printed in the United States of America

Contents

Preface

Why did I write a book about pharmaceutical sales?

There are lots of answers, but the biggest one is that many trainers and other pharmaceutical sales professionals have *asked* for it. And I know that I would have *loved* to have read a book like this when I first evaluated pharmaceutical selling as a career option.

The fact is, although pharmaceutical sales is one of the most sought after and rewarding careers in American industry, many representatives sort of stumble into it. Too many representatives begin their careers with little or no framework of what a pharmaceutical sales career is really all about. There is no *Pharmaceutical Selling 101* course in any university curriculum that I know of. For many representatives, the first exposure to a possible career in the industry is a 3″ x 5″ ad in the Sunday newspaper.

With some careful searching, you'll find a handful of books that promote the benefits of pharmaceutical selling and that walk you through the ins and outs of resume preparation and job interviews. Others tell you something about basic selling skills and profile typical sales calls. All of these books are worthwhile in many respects, and I've included a list in the appendix.

To date, however, I have yet to discover a definitive presentation on pharmaceutical selling for the beginner or novice; one which tells you clearly and concisely exactly what this career is all about on a day-to-day basis while capturing the essence of the prescription drug marketplace in the new century.

In my opinion (and according to many others who encouraged me to write this book), there's no publication out there that provides you with the "jump start" that I think a representative should have—and that all sales managers love to see— before drawing that first paycheck.

That is exactly what I hope this book will do for you.

As you'll learn, the book's title—*Be Brief. Be Bright. Be Gone.*—reflects my personal selling philosophy. It also candidly reflects the wishes of many of the tens of thousands of physicians and other health-care professionals who interact with sales representatives every day. These individuals expect sales representatives to:

- *Be brief.* Keep your sales presentations short and to the point.
- *Be bright.* Understand your product and its clinical context.
- *Be gone.* Respect your customer's time.

Throughout my sales career, I practiced this philosophy and it worked very well for me. I've tried to capture the same philosophy in the text. I hope you'll discover that I'm brief, and that I'm bright. And. although I'll "be gone" in a sense when you put this book down, I hope you'll keep it as a permanent reference source to help keep you on track throughout your pharmaceutical sales career.

David Currier
January 2001

A word to managers and sales trainers who read this book

I know that the directive, "Be gone," probably flies in the face of advice you would like your representatives to hear. You probably prefer telling them that one of their objectives is to get as much face time as possible in front of physicians and that my "Be gone" directive runs counter to good selling techniques.

I do not disagree with this position. It was always one of my objectives as a sales representative to spend as much time as possible with every physician whom I met. Twenty minutes with a physician is usually more productive than two minutes.

*However, I found that I had to **earn** the privilege of spending that kind of time with a doctor. And one way that I earned that privilege was to make it absolutely clear to them early on that I respected their time. This is why "Be gone" was an important tactic for me when I first met a doctor.*

I discovered that if I was brief, bright, and gone on the first two or three visits, most doctors seemed to think, "Hey, this guy gets it. He knows how valuable my time is and never tries to overstay his welcome as some of these other reps do. I think I'll spend a little more time with him next time he's here."

Sure enough, after a few weeks or months of "Be gone" calls, I noted that most doctors were spending a lot more time with me. This allowed my strategy to evolve into one of, "Be brief. Be bright. And be gone when appropriate."

I am convinced that this "3 Be's" philosophy contributed significantly to the success I enjoyed in the field.

Introduction

About me. About you. About this book.

About me

As a general rule, it's of questionable etiquette for sales representatives to talk too much about themselves, but I do want to provide you with an understanding of why I think I am qualified to write this book:

- I am an experienced and successful pharmaceutical sales representative. For nearly ten years, I worked for the pharmaceutical company whose sales force has been consistently rated highest by physicians. I have promoted prescription drugs in many therapeutic categories (allergy, arthritis, cardiovascular, endocrine, psychiatric, etc.) to many types of physicians in a variety of settings—from rural primary care physicians (PCPs) to highly educated academic specialists; from solo-practice doctors' offices to community hospitals to large teaching institutions to huge multi-state managed care organizations.
- I have received numerous sales awards and tens of thousands of dollars in bonuses for exceptional short-and long-term sales performance.
- I have spent several years as a pharmaceutical sales training manager—from teaching new hires to helping experienced representatives develop their careers.

- In the mid-1990s, I was intimately involved at the management level in the largest sales force expansion in the history of the industry, as a coach and mentor to hundreds of representatives-to-be.
- My experience has provided me with expertise in the three critical areas required for sales success—selling skills (*how* you sell), clinical understanding (*what* you sell), and market knowledge (*where* you sell).

I have consulted with many of the nation's leading pharmaceutical companies in the development of effective training programs in all three of these essential areas. Currently I work for one of the world's premier biotechnology companies providing training in the areas of selling and coaching, key account management, and career development programs.

About you

Enough about me.

What about you?

Do you think you have what it takes to be successful in pharmaceutical sales?

You may have heard stories about some of the perks–the company car, product-launch events at the lavish resorts, award trips and cash bonuses, the outstanding compensation packages. All true.

But what about this…

Have you heard about the 14-hour days? The 4 a.m. visits to emergency rooms to try to catch five minutes with a tough-to-see physician? About the fact that you have to get up to speed in a few weeks on clinical knowledge that takes physicians months to master?

Have you heard about the resistance you'll typically encounter on a daily basis? About the doctors who refuse to speak with you—and whose receptionists, in a not-too-friendly manner, are all to happy to show you the door?

Are you aware of how cut-throat the competition can be? How managed care can deal you and your company out of millions of dollars in business at the stroke of a pen? How disgruntled patients, physicians, and managed care administrators can become when they discover the cost of your company's "breakthrough" product?

You'll run into all of these issues in the field, which means that you must possess a number of essential character traits to ensure your long-term success. For example, you must be:

- *Goal-oriented*—You must develop specific sales goals that you are expected to meet. People who set and work toward goals are more successful than those who do not.
- *Organized*—This means that you must be able to plan your months, weeks, and days, sometimes down to the hour; and you must have your car and "bag" (rep lingo for "briefcase") arranged so that you can find key items on a moment's notice.
- *Resilient*—You will encounter resistance more often than you'd like, but you will learn to bounce back quickly in order to capture the next piece of business.
- *Optimistic*—This is an ideal career for those who view life with a "can-do" attitude.
- *Assertive*—You very often must leave your comfort zone to ask a doctor to prescribe your product. If you don't, you can be certain that a competitive representative will.
- *Outgoing*—You are *always* meeting new people…doctors, nurses, office staff, pharmacists, colleagues in your company; it's up to *you* to take the initiative and generate goodwill for yourself an your company.

If this sounds like you, then you are reading the perfect publication to help prepare you for a career in pharmaceutical sales.

About this book

This book features 11 chapters designed to provide useful information about a career in pharmaceutical sales. It is designed for anyone considering a career in pharmaceutical sales and for those who have been newly hired by pharmaceutical sales organizations.

Here are brief previews of the chapters:

Chapter 1: A Great Career Choice summarizes the advantages and rewards that come with a successful career in pharmaceuticals.

Chapter 2: The Drawbacks (Just So You Know) takes an honest look at some of the reasons why some people *don't* consider pharmaceuticals as the ideal career.

Chapter 3: Getting Hired outlines the typical hiring process and provides tips on how to land a job in pharmaceutical selling.

Chapter 4: Getting Started provides an overview of the training you will complete as a newly-hired representative.

Chapter 5: Getting Organized acquaints you with some of the basics about organizing your office, your car, and your time.

Chapter 6: Meet Your Customers profiles physicians and other medical personnel whom you'll visit on a daily basis. This chapter also takes a look at hospital selling.

Chapter 7: Basic Selling Skills covers some of the skills that are essential for communicating and establishing rapport with your customers.

Chapter 8: The Sales Call walks you through the "typical" pharmaceutical sales call. (I put quotes around the word because there is no "typical" call in this industry.)

Chapter 9: Supporting the Sales Call summarizes the tools and methods you'll use to back up your product presentations.

Chapter 10: The Managed Care Marketplace provides need-to-know information about the market in which you'll be selling.

Chapter 11: Top 10 Ways to Jump-start Your Pharmaceutical Sales Career concludes the book with the top ten techniques that worked for me when I sold pharmaceuticals in the field.

The book concludes with and a brief bibliography, internet resources, and a representative list of major US pharmaceutical companies with their addresses, home office telephone numbers, and website locations.

Chapter 1

A *Great* Career Choice

Why do tens of thousands of people apply for pharmaceutical selling jobs every year, and why do many of those who make the first cut stay in pharmaceutical sales for decades? The profession *must* have something going for it.

It sure does. Lots of great things…starting with money.

Compensation

Consider the monetary rewards alone. How would you like to generate $30,000 to $50,000—or even more—in annual bonuses *on top of* a salary that already puts you in the top 20% of all wage earners?

It can happen, even as early as your second or third year in the field.

Compensation packages vary dramatically in pharmaceutical selling, but virtually all companies provide a base salary plus performance-based commissions and bonuses. Base salaries for entry-level representatives typically run from the mid thirties to mid forties. In addition, commissions are often paid quarterly and are based on prescription volume in your territory, usually by product.

Most companies structure bonus incentives into their compensation agreements, so if a particular product does well in your territory, and you beat your "numbers" (your sales targets) by a certain amount, you can expect anywhere from $5,000 to $50,000 annually in bonuses and commissions. One company (which, it should be noted, pays significantly lower base salaries than the industry norm) recently paid out bonuses in the range of $30,000 per *quarter.*

Compensation varies by region, too. Salaries are relatively consistent throughout a company's field sales force. However, representatives who service major metropolitan areas heavily populated by teaching hospitals and large physician group practices often have greater bonus earnings potential than representatives who service lightly populated rural areas. (Keep in mind that the representative who lives in a rural area may enjoy certain lifestyle and cost-of-living benefits not readily available to the urban representative.)

Note, too, that many companies offer special incentives for top performers. For example, at some companies it's possible to win all-expense-paid trips for you and your significant other to tropical paradises where you stay and dine at world-class resorts, golf on tour-quality courses, and shop 'til you drop. Every pharmaceutical company takes care of its top performers.

Career advancement

Here's something else to consider…Many senior management, marketing, and other highly sought after and well rewarded positions in large pharmaceutical companies are filled by those who were successful in the field.

If you are successful in field sales, the potential rewards are equally compelling whether you consider staying in sales or climbing the corporate ladder. Career advancement opportunities exist in sales management, account management, marketing and product management, and training management.

If you are good and possess the requisite management—and political—skills, you can write your own ticket.

Benefits to others

In recent decades, the pharmaceutical industry has been one of the crown jewels in American industry. Public academic centers certainly have made contributions to medical research, but many of the prescription drugs that are enhancing and prolonging human life were funded and developed by private industry.

Major pharmaceutical companies invest billions of dollars a year in research and development, an average of about 20% of total revenues per company. That's good for patients and society, good for the industry—and good for anyone who is out there successfully promoting pharmaceuticals to healthcare professionals.

To me, one of the most rewarding aspects about working in pharmaceutical sales is that you help improve the quality of life for thousands of men, women, and children.

Here's an example of what I mean. One of the best experiences of my professional life occurred when I called on an internist at a community hospital. After visiting him for over a year, one day he waved me in to his office from the waiting room, invited me to sit down, and said, "Dave, I want to thank you for all the information and product samples you have given me. I'm going to introduce you to a woman who has tried and failed with a number of antidepressant drugs. Because of you and the information you have provided, I prescribed your company's product. It has really turned her life around."

Needless to say, I was walking on air after that encounter. I am confident that most experienced representatives in the field today have similar human interest stories to share. These stories are exceptionally gratifying and can be powerful motivators for representatives.

An education in itself

Think, too, in terms of the educational advantages you enjoy as your pharmaceutical sales career evolves. You have countless opportunities to study, learn, and communicate about some highly advanced clinical information and about how the American healthcare system works.

You will learn all of this in your product training programs, by attending seminars and conferences, and through your day-to-day interactions with physicians and other medical professionals.

I remember riding with a representative who was modeling sales calls for me prior to my formal initiation to field sales. I had a very difficult time understanding his interactions with physicians. To think I would be able to learn, understand, and talk about stuff like glomerular filtration rate and neurotransmitter re-uptake inhibition was very intimidating. But I overcame the fear factor and discovered medical science to be an exhilarating field to be involved with.

Great people

Sales representatives get to meet, interact, and develop rewarding relationships with fascinating people. People who work in the healthcare field (doctors, nurses, physician assistants, etc.) are some of the most interesting and dedicated people you will ever meet. They love and care for their patients, and most are willing to share their knowledge with you.

It's true that a very small percentage of doctors do suffer from the "Ivory Tower" syndrome and sometimes display their arrogance toward sales professionals, but most are not like this. Doctors are considered to be among the most well educated professional in our society, and they do lead lives outside of the office. They hold a lot of interesting opinions on many subjects. And most of them are often willing to share stories about kids and family, hobbies, vacation travel, and the success of the local sports teams.

Investment potential

Here's another reason why selling pharmaceuticals can be rewarding: As an investment sector, the pharmaceutical industry has been instrumental in driving key stock indexes for several years.

If you are employed by a publicly traded pharmaceutical company, chances are your compensation package will include stock options. Pharmaceutical stocks, at least in recent years, have represented a great long-term investment, and the future looks bright in this regard.

As a rule, older people have more health problems than younger people, so with the aging of the Baby Boom generation, the market for pharmaceuticals should continue to grow. And it looks like many of the big pharmaceutical companies will continue launching blockbuster drugs that enhance and extend the quality of life—from sexual dysfunction drugs to products that effectively treat chronic diseases such as rheumatoid arthritis and certain types of cancer.

In short, you can be reasonably confident that there will always be jobs for pharmaceutical sales representatives.

*   *   *   *   *

So now you know all about the substantial benefits you can accrue by promoting pharmaceuticals for a major corporation.

Sounds like a very attractive career, doesn't it?

Chapter 2

The Drawbacks
(Just So You Know)

Every career has some potential disadvantages, and pharmaceutical sales is no exception. I feel obligated to acquaint you with some of the less-than-positive issues that come with the turf. I don't want to make pharmaceutical sales sound *too* inviting. Selling pharmaceuticals poses some significant challenges for every representative. You work in a highly competitive—some might even say cut-throat—environment. I don't want you to try it only to wind up frustrated, disappointed, out of a job, and upset at me for leading you on.

So let's take an honest look at some of the major challenges that all representatives encounter in their careers.

Not an easy job

The bottom line is that the job of being a pharmaceutical representative is not an easy one and the hard work starts right away, with your initial training. Very often, you must spend weeks at a time away from friends and family. You might even find yourself living in a hotel with a roommate whose snoring keeps you awake throughout the night.

Training managers expect you to learn the equivalent of an entire semester's worth of highly scientific clinical information in a very short amount of time (and you probably think you spent your last all-nighter in college!).

"No problem," you say. "I can handle that."

Well, the difference between college and the high-pressure world of pharmaceutical sales industry is enormous in terms of the expectations of the individuals who control your destiny. In college you generally went into a lecture, sat down, picked up a blue book and a pencil, and the information flowed out of your brain, down your arm, and onto the paper…where it probably stayed forever.

Pharmaceutical training is a lot different. Not only do you encounter a huge amount of technical information, but you are actually expected to *know* it, inside and out, backward and forward. And believe me, there will come a time in the field when you *must* know it, because some physician will probably question you about it when you least expect it.

In college, you can probably get away with a few C's every now and then. In training for a pharmaceutical sales job, anything under 80% is often considered failing. Get a couple of C's at a major pharmaceutical company, and you may be out of a job.

Not only that, but you are expected to *articulate* your knowledge so that it makes sense when your manager—or a highly educated physician—asks you about it!

As you can see, a fairly high level of academic acumen is required for this particular career.

Break-in period

After completing your initial "new hire" training (which can last anywhere from three to six months), you must make it through your first year in the field, which presents a number of challenges. Actually, as you'll learn in training, every challenge represents an opportunity, so let's call them *opportunities.*

Normally, the first year in your territory is considered your break-in period. Most new representatives are in survival mode during that time, and after about a year, they either make it or begin a new career search.

It's common for rookie representatives to get lost—literally and figuratively—in their new and unfamiliar surroundings. Lost, in the sense that you may not know your way around from one physician practice to another. (You'll need to take care to avoid accidents when driving and map-reading simultaneously.)

Then, when you finally reach your destination, if you are unskilled at opening calls, doctors may show you little respect; nor will the office "gatekeepers," the receptionists who occupy positions of power behind those glass windows. Selling—or, more precisely, attempting to sell—is tough to do when few medical personnel take any time to talk with you.

It's especially no fun when a doctor decides to test your mettle by telling you that your product is lousy, causes all kinds of serious side effects, and maybe even kills people—when in reality he or she is a product champion who prescribes your product on a daily basis.

I am not making this up. It happens.

12-to 14-hour days

For the successful pharmaceutical sales representative, 12-to 14-hour days are not unusual. Of course, you won't be calling on doctors during all of those hours. You will spend dozens of hours each week planning your calls, writing call reports, updating your training, preparing expense reports, reading publications and e-mails, and attending sales and marketing meetings.

That's not all. You're often required to work many evenings running "programs," which are educational events for physicians and nurses.

You'll also log many hours in your home office, and you'll maintain a storage unit full of product samples and marketing supplies.

Daytime hours are generally filled with office calls, one after another, all day long. You'll drive and drive and drive and drive. Like me, you may find yourself standing in slush up to your shins at 6:30 p.m. on a Friday night in February looking for samples in your trunk with two hours of driving ahead of you to get home. Also, like me, you may find yourself melting in your business suit when it's 98° and humid while lugging half a dozen pizzas across a couple of city blocks. Every experienced representative can tell you "war stories" like these.

It can get pretty lonely out there too. If you enjoy office camaraderie and constant interaction with others, reconsider pharmaceutical sales. For many hours, it's you and your favorite talk show host, classic rock, or the latest training cassette. When you're in the field, you are often very much alone.

Making numbers

Selling is selling. While you're driving around your territory with a carload of literature and product samples, you've got to make your "numbers"—or budget, or sales quota, or whatever your company calls it.

Occasionally, you can coast, especially if you promote a product that has a unique and well-known clinical advantage, a medicine that "sells itself," so to speak (there are precious few of these). But you must be aware at all times that your job is to generate prescriptions. And you will find out very quickly if you are not producing more prescriptions to meet your ever-expanding quota.

Your district manager is your coach and mentor, but keep in mind that he must follow your every move and routinely check reports on your performance, doctor by doctor, hospital by hospital. Your performance is also being compared with that of your colleagues in your district, your region, and your division. Making 100% of your sales quota for each of the products you are selling is great unless others average 115%. In that case, 100% may not be enough.

Competitive pressure

Intense competition in the industry adds another challenge. Maybe you did well in college and in other jobs and enjoy a high level of self-confidence. That's great, but if you are not prepared to take some "hits" every now and then, pharmaceutical selling can shatter one's self-esteem overnight.

Most everyone in the field has at least a four-year college degree, and many representatives hold masters degrees in business administration or perhaps in a biological science. You can assume that most other representatives are just as savvy, intelligent, and determined as you are. This is because pharmaceutical companies hire only the best—the cream of the crop. So, as bright as you are, you are just one among the 50,000 or more representatives across the country who are making sales calls every day.

Consider this: During a divisional expansion in which I was involved, my company received approximately 60,000 resumes for *five hundred* open positions. You may have better luck applying to and getting into Harvard, Yale, or Stanford than landing a sales slot at a major pharmaceutical company.

Consider this, too: Countless pharmaceutical products are considered to be "me too" products. For example, most major companies in the cardiovascular marketplace sell blood pressure drugs that are extremely close in chemical composition, mechanism of action, side effects, dosing, and cost. So part of your job may be to convince doctors that your company's drug is better, when, in the eyes of your customer, there is little or no difference at all.

*   *   *   *   *

As I said, it is not an easy job.

A lot of people try pharmaceutical sales and give up because they are frustrated by one or more of the items covered in this chapter. I don't want this to happen to you. If you're serious about selling pharmaceuticals, take some time to think about how these issues apply.

Chapter 3

Getting Hired

Keep in mind that, when you first apply for a job in pharmaceutical sales, you are simply one among perhaps hundreds of individuals applying for each opening.

My experience suggests that pharmaceutical companies have fairly similar qualifications in order to land a job as a representative. Virtually all of them will require a BA or BS with a grade point average no lower than 3.0. Some say no lower than 3.5. Some companies prefer prior sales experience, but most companies will train qualified, motivated applicants.

As is the case with most professional job openings, evaluators quickly dismiss as many as 90% of applicants because they are unqualified, fail to follow instructions regarding the submission of materials, or present poorly prepared cover letters and resumes.

That leaves roughly 10%—or perhaps even fewer—who are invited for an interview.

Consider then that for every job opening, more than a hundred may apply, ten or so will have interviews—and only one will get the job. This chapter will tell you how to find jobs in the industry and how to narrow the odds in your favor in an interview to ensure that *you* are that one-in-a-hundred individual who lands the job.

Finding the job openings

Your first step in securing a position as a pharmaceutical sales representative requires you to find out which companies are hiring. This is easy to do, thanks to the internet. Simply locate a company's website and on the home page you will usually find a bar or icon for "Employment" or "Job Listings." Click again and you'll find a list of sales openings, often listed by geography.

Most companies post sales openings in the employment listings of major metropolitan newspapers. The best newspaper source is usually the Sunday employment listings. Recently, the Boston *Globe* has run a multipage section devoted exclusively to the pharmaceutical industry. On one Sunday, several dozen sales jobs were advertised by an impressive cross-section of companies.

Some companies contract out the screening process, so check the listings of executive recruiting firms, too.

If you are still in college, check the bulletin board and web page of your school's placement office for scheduled recruiter visits.

One of the best proactive strategies to land a job in pharmaceutical sales is to visit several physician offices. Ask the receptionists to provide you with the names and numbers of as many pharmaceutical representatives as possible. You may even be able to obtain photocopies of business cards of representatives who routinely call on the practice.

Then, research several companies (company's websites are the best starting points), target ten of them, and call the local representative for each targeted company. Explain how you obtained the representative's name and number and sell yourself on the telephone.

Even if there are no current job openings, ask the representative where you should mail your resume. Even better, schedule a lunch with the representative (on you), during which you will obtain information about the company and the job. You may even be able to present your resume to the representative and ask him or her forward your resume to the right person.

This method is a great way to "network" yourself into a company. If you are hired, chances are, the representative will get a finder's fee (which is usually considerably lower than the fee that the company would pay to a recruiting firm).

The job interview

When you are accepted for an interview at a major pharmaceutical company you will probably meet with several key people in the organization including:
- your future district manager (DM)
- a regional manager (RM)
- a human resources (or personnel) specialist

You may also meet with other people in the sales organization, including a territory sales representative, who may be your future team member in the field.

At most companies, you must complete a series of interviews before you are hired. These include:
- a *screening interview*, which is designed to identify the top candidates from those who submitted reasonably acceptable resumes. This interview may be conducted by a human resource specialist or a representative from a recruiting firm. This type of interview is sometimes done via telephone.
- a *first interview*, usually conducted by a district manager—your first chance to sell yourself to your future supervisor.
- a *follow-up interview*, indicating that the company considers you to be a serious candidate. This interview may be conducted by a panel, including the district manager, a regional manager,

and possibly a product specialist (if you will be assigned to a product group).

- a *final interview*, suggesting that you are very close to receiving a job offer. This provides you and the supervisory team with one more opportunity to ask questions about each other and, perhaps, to discuss a compensation package, a potential start date, and so on.

Your interview represents your first selling experience at a pharmaceutical company. In this situation, you are selling yourself, and you sell yourself much in the same manner as you would sell any other commodity.

Your most important strategy is to identify a personal advantage that makes you unique among the other candidates who have been chosen for interviews. A unique advantage might include:

- sales success at another pharmaceutical company
- sales success in another industry
- experience in nursing or another clinical field (e.g., laboratory science, nutrition, radiology)
- a degree in clinical pharmacology
- experience as a hospital or retail pharmacist
- outstanding academic success in the life sciences or business
- a pre-medical education
- proof that you are a "quick study," as demonstrated by your ability to adapt to other positions that you may have held

Like many employers, pharmaceutical companies prefer experience, so a successful selling tour at another pharmaceutical company will often provide you with an advantage. Of course, if that is your background, you probably wouldn't be reading this book, so try to identify one or more of the above characteristics that apply to you.

I will say that I have trained many successful representatives who entered the industry directly from college. Actually, several companies don't want previous pharmaceutical sales experience–they prefer to train you "their" way.

Interviewers will look for qualities from your past experience and performance in sales, your academic success, and examples of initiative.

Obviously, it is to your advantage to present yourself in the best possible light at every interview in terms of personal appearance and demeanor. This book will not provide specific interviewing tips. Anne Clayton's *Insight into a Career in Pharmaceutical Sales* features a comprehensive chapter on interviewing, including 50 common interviewer questions and suggested response techniques, plus questions that you can ask the interviewer about the company and the position.

The rep ride

At some time during the interview process, you may be asked to go on a "rep ride." This is your opportunity to spend a half-day or full day with a territory representative and see exactly how a pharmaceutical representative performs his or her daily selling activities.

During your rep ride, you may decide that a pharmaceutical sales really isn't for you after all. On the other hand, you may be impressed by the fast-paced academic discussions, the excitement, and the "adrenaline rush" that accompanies many sales interactions.

Use the time spent with a representative to ask as many questions as you can about the career. You'll normally have plenty of time between calls to accomplish this.

Of course, while you are assessing the work of the territory representative, his or her objective is to assess your enthusiasm and capabilities and to report back to the DM. So be on your best behavior. Essentially, a territory representative is simply looking for someone who will make a good teammate, someone who is genuinely interested in the job and asks good questions. (As you'll learn later, asking good questions is one of the most important skills a pharmaceutical sales representative can possess.)

The ride is designed to be informal. Relax. Be yourself. Stay politically correct. If you hear a term you don't understand, such as "pharmacokinetics" or "formulary," ask the representative for a definition (never during a call, of course). On a repride, there are no "stupid" questions.

I recall my rep ride vividly. I remember that I didn't understand any of the clinical language that the representative used—he may as well have been speaking Greek or Russian–but I loved what I saw. For me, there was no looking back.

So let's assume that you survived the hiring process (which can take up to six or eight weeks). You were selected from among more than a hundred candidates, signed the employment contract, and agreed to report to work on a certain date.

What should you expect during your first few weeks at your new job?

Chapter 4

Getting Started

It's your first—or maybe second—day at work. You've completed all the human resources paperwork, selected your insurance coverage, read the employee handbook, and discovered the locations of the cafeteria and the rest rooms.

Now it's time to meet the people you'll work with and to begin training for your first day of selling.

Meet the sales team

You've already heard me mention the "sales team." That's because, even though you work independently and manage all or part of a territory, you are definitely part of a team. Without effective teamwork, neither you nor your company will achieve maximum sales potential. So let's look at the team.

The Geography of Pharmaceutical Selling

Pharmaceutical selling has its own geographical terminology that is common among most companies. Most pharmaceutical sales organizations are structured according to geography, as follows:

- *Headquarters: Executive-level sales managers (e.g., the vice president of sales as well as directors and support staff) usually work out of corporate headquarters. National account managers (NAMs), who sell to large managed care organizations (MCOs) and pharmacy benefit management companies (PBMs), also typically work at corporate headquarters. Other professionals you will meet are product managers who are part of the company's marketing department. They are charged with orchestrating the overall strategy that you implement in the marketplace.*
- *Regions: Most sales organizations divide the country into five to ten geographic regions, each of which is supervised by a regional manager (RM). Typical regions might be "New England," "Mid-Atlantic," "Mid-West," "Southeast," etc.*
- *Districts: Each region features several districts, and each district is supervised by a district manager (DM). For example, a New England sales region might be divided into separate districts for Maine, New Hampshire, Vermont, and Rhode Island. Heavily populated states such as Massachusetts and Connecticut are typically split into several districts. Massachusetts, for example, might be split into two or three districts in the eastern part of the state (in and around Greater Boston) with separate districts for the central and western parts of the state.*
- *Territories: Finally, each district includes from 8 to 12 territories. Territories are staffed by territory representatives (which is the job that you will probably apply for). Some representatives cover a territory by*

themselves. Other territories may be staffed by several representatives (for example, some who call exclusively on hospitals and other who call on physician offices; and some companies assign representatives to promote different products within the same territory).

At most companies, the sales team consists of:
- territory representatives
- specialty, hospital, and institutional representatives
- district manager (DM)
- regional manager (RM)
- national account manager

Territory representative. The heart of the team—the group that interacts with customers on a daily basis—is based in your district and usually consists of 8 to 12 territory representatives[*], each of whom has a specific geographical territory to cover.

Square mileage depends on the part of the country in which the representative works. If your territory is Montana, you may "own" the whole state—or maybe half the state and half of Idaho, too.

(If your territory is Montana, you will want to have a good audio system in your car and stock up on your favorite CD's and Books on Tape. You will also have plenty of time to listen to the collection of audiocassette training tapes provided by your company.)

If, on the other hand, your territory is metropolitan Boston or Chicago, it may be possible to park your car in a downtown garage all day and complete all your calls on foot among the city's hospitals, clinics, and physician group practices.

---

[*] Some companies refer to territory representatives as "professional sales representatives," or "PSRs."

Regardless of how a company configures its territories, each team member is assigned approximately the same number of physicians to call on.

Specialty, hospital, and niche representatives. Specialty and hospital representatives sell exclusively to niche markets. Specialty representatives are trained to sell to specific physician specialists, such as cardiologists, endocrinologists, or oncologists. Hospital representatives (or institutional representatives, at some companies) call exclusively on hospitals. Institutional representatives may also call on Veterans Administration (VA) hospitals, as well as nursing homes, home health-care agencies, and rehabilitation centers. Normally, representatives who sell to hospitals and other institutions have been promoted from the ranks of territory representatives.

District manager (DM). Territory representatives report to a district manager. His or her responsibility is to coach and mentor territory representatives. DMs also ensure that each representative is making his or her required calls and is on track to achieve monthly, quarterly, semi-annual, and annual sales goals.

The DM regularly conducts in-person or telephone conferences with territory representatives as a group and on an individual basis. The DM often arranges for district-wide training programs and may deliver the training at workshops and seminars.

DMs often accompany representatives in the field to observe selling techniques, reinforce good selling behaviors, and critique areas that may require improvement. Some DMs may manage a few special accounts, such as local managed care organizations (MCOs).

The DM is the sales representative's primary point of contact to and from the rest of the corporation. Most DMs are former territory representatives who earned promotions and are very much in tune with day-to-day selling requirements. A DM is a very important resource for the territory representative.

DMs have a challenging job. They are generally "on call" 24 hours a day, 7 days a week for their reps. They must also endure an enormous amount of paperwork and are responsible for a great deal of logistical planning and reporting up through channels.

Regional Manager (RM). District managers report to a regional manager. The regional manager sets the strategy for a region and monitors sales activity in each district under his or her supervision.

In today's healthcare marketplace, healthcare delivery systems are often regionalized. This means that healthcare payment systems—and probably policies relating to physician prescribing and prescription reimbursement—are different in the Pacific states than they are, say, in the Southeast or Upper Midwest. The regional manager must be in tune with these issues and develop a region-wide sales and marketing strategy that is tailored to the specific needs of his or her geography.

National account manager (NAM). In recent years, a relatively new type of manager has become prominent in pharmaceutical sales—the national account manager, or NAM. The NAM's primary role is to negotiate product purchasing contracts with major MCOs and giant pharmacy benefit managers (PBMs*).

---

*PBMs are large nationwide corporations that manage prescription drug benefit programs on behalf of managed care organizations (or, in some cases, for large employers that contract directly for drug benefits). PBMs design and manage drug formularies, arrange for MCO contracts with retail pharmacies, coordinate drug reimbursement, and manage prescription data for MCOs.

Variations of sales organization structure

A pharmaceutical company may feature two or more selling divisions, each with its own proprietary portfolio of drugs to sell. Often, these divisions are based on therapeutic category.

For example, a company may have a sales division for cardiovascular products, another for infectious disease agents (antibiotics), and another for injectables (such as vaccines). Thus, it is possible that three different representatives from the same company might visit the same physician's office in a single day, promoting three different sets of products.

Companies may also create separate sales forces according to targeted customer groups. For example, one sales force may call only on primary care physicians, another on specialists (e.g., cardiologists, endocrinologists, or OB-GYNs), and another on hospital-based physicians.

What do you need to know?—*Everything* (it seems)

Your first assignment following your hiring as a new sales representative is to read. You will receive volumes, several weeks' worth, in fact.

In fact, you might think of your first few weeks on the job as a huge cramming course in which you must learn about

- general medical terminology
- anatomy and physiology
- clinical pharmacology

And all of this is merely prelude to a series of workshops and training sessions where you'll listen to lectures, watch videos, participate in role plays, play competitive games, and examine case studies—all in preparation for your first sales call.

Very often, your training materials are provided in the form of home study programs. I'll never forget my excitement when the Federal Express driver delivered the first package I ever received from my former employer. I felt like a kid at Christmastime. I opened the oversized carton, extracted several books (including a hefty medical dictionary) and said to myself, "This is going to be great!"

Then I read the cover letter, which informed me that I had five days to read the material (it looked like at least a month's worth of reading), after which I would have to complete a series of examinations. I was reminded of the scene from the movie *The Paper Chase,* where several law students, trying to prepare for finals, check into a motel, throw out the TV, lock the door, and don't emerge for a week. That's about what happened with me.

In some situations, you may take exams over the phone by providing touch-tone responses to pre-recorded questions. In other situations, the company will put you up at a hotel and you may take the exams in a hotel conference room or at a company office suite.

Product learning systems

Assuming that you pass the exams, you will then be presented with at least one product "learning system"—but probably more than one. These learning systems are professionally developed by companies that create training materials exclusively for pharmaceutical companies. They provide "need to know" information (and a lot more) about diseases and products that treat them.

The typical learning system consists of a series of three-ring binders or 8 ½" x 11" perfect-bound books that cover:

- disease background (prevalence of a disease, its cost to society, the demand for therapy)
- anatomy and physiology specific to the disease (e.g., the cardiovascular system for a blood pressure drug)

- signs, symptoms, and diagnostic procedures
- current treatment alternatives
- product information (usually a walk-through of the package insert [see box], plus analyses of key clinical studies that support the product's advantages)
- how to sell the product (target audience profiles, key promotional messages, features and benefits, competitive product profiles, and anticipated questions and objections)

All or part of some learning systems may be produced on CD-ROM, audiocassette, or video.

What's a "package insert"?

A package insert (PI) is a small, multifold informational sheet that accompanies prescription products to physician offices and retail pharmacies. The text is printed at about the same size as the footnote text that appears in this book, maybe even smaller.

The federal Food and Drug Administration (FDA) requires that pharmaceutical manufacturers provide PI data for all prescription drug products.

PIs feature highly detailed clinical information about the product including chemical makeup, mechanism of action, clinical pharmacology, pharmacokinetics, indications, contraindications, clinical study summaries, adverse event profiles, warnings and precautions, drug interactions, dosing and administration, and packaging.

PI data on any product is available to consumers upon request at retail prescription counters whenever a prescription is dispensed. Anyone can view PI data by consulting the Physician's Desk Reference (usually referred to as the PDR) or viewing product information at drug manufacturer websites.

The PDR, which is updated annually, is available at bookstores and public libraries in reference sections. Pharmaceutical companies often provide PDRs for their sales representatives because the PDR is the best single source of information about competitive products.

PI data is often too complex for a layperson to understand. Consequently, many companies have begun creating "Patient Product Information" sheets that present need-to-know information for patients in a reader-friendly manner.

The number of learning systems you must read depends upon the number of products you will sell. Most representatives sell a "portfolio" or "suite" of from three to five medications.

For sales representatives in most industries, promoting just three to five products probably sounds like a piece of cake. But I have some sobering news for aspiring pharmaceutical sales representatives. Three to five products represent an enormous workload, even for the most savvy of representatives, especially if each product is in a different therapeutic category.

Consider this: For every product that you sell, you must be intimately familiar with anatomy and physiology of the specific body systems in question (e.g., the heart and circulatory system for cardiovascular products). You must also learn all about the pathophysiology[*] of the disease in question, diagnostic methods, therapeutic alternatives, and so on.

---

[*] Pathophysiology refers to the functional changes that occur within the body in response to a particular disease. For example, diabetes is often accompanied by renal (kidney) failure. Therefore, if you promote a diabetes drug, you would be required to learn about the anatomy and physiology of renal system, as well as the changes that occur in the renal system when diabetes is present.

For every product you sell, you must virtually memorize the PI, as well as the PIs of the leading competitive products, including the clinical studies related to your product and studies related to competitive products. (You will learn more about clinical studies in Chapter 9.)

Sounds like a lot to learn, doesn't it?

Guess what…There's more. Lots more.

Know your market

After you work your way through the product learning systems, you'll probably spend a considerable amount of time learning about the healthcare marketplace—the business environment in which you will sell your products.

Not too long ago, pharmaceutical sales professionals rarely learned—or cared—about the healthcare "marketplace." That's because physicians received virtually all of their compensation via the traditional fee-for-service method and made virtually all prescribing decisions autonomously. You sold the doc, you sold the 'script,'** and that was it. It didn't matter whether you promoted your product in Portland, Maine, or Portland, Oregon. The routine was the same.

In recent years, however, managed care has become the dominant driver in healthcare decision-making, and managed care wields enormous influence regarding the ways in which physicians manage their practices, diagnose and treat patients, and prescribe medications.

Today, it takes literally months, if not years, to understand managed care, integrated healthcare systems, physician group practices, pharmacy benefit management, clinical practice guidelines, disease management,

---

** "Script" is sales rep jargon for "prescription."

physician compensation management, risk-bearing strategies, and dozens of other managed care concepts. And just when you think you've mastered all the issues, a new generation of managed care comes along, which means that you advance along a completely new learning curve.

In short, it is never enough to simply understand your product's clinical issues and how the product can benefit patients. You *must* be able to understand managed care and the key business issues confronting the physicians in your territory.

It would be very embarrassing, for example, to call on Dr. Jones to promote "Product X" only to have Dr. Jones tell you, "You're wasting your time. I can't prescribe Product X because it's not on formulary [the approved drug list] at ABC Health Plan."

When you sell in a managed care environment, you'll need to understand a broad range of contemporary health economics issues—capitation, disease management, formularies, clinical practice guidelines, outcomes, quality-of-life studies, integrated delivery systems, gate-keeper physicians, pharmacy benefit management, three-tiered copayments, and a whole lot more.

Managed care selling also demands that you memorize and be able to define a dizzying array of acronyms: not only MCO and PBM (to which you have already been introduced in this chapter), but AAPCC, DRG, DUE, DUR, HEDIS, IPA, NCQA, P&T, PCP, PHO, PMPM, PPO, QALY, UCR, and dozens of others.

You'll receive an introduction to managed care selling in Chapter 10. You'll learn much more in the managed care training manuals, audio-cassettes, workshops, and case studies provided by your company. The rest—perhaps most of what you'll learn—will come from your experience in the field and what you learn from physicians, nurses, office managers, and pharmacists.

Selling skills

You're still not done.

The last—and probably the most critical phase of your initial training relates to selling skills. These are the interpersonal skills required to successfully complete business interactions with your customers. These training programs, which usually feature a mix of text, video, and interactive role plays, typically address:

- communication skills
- negotiation skills
- the structure of a sales call (opening, probing to identify needs, matching features and benefits to needs, handling questions and objections, closing for a commitment)

Many companies prepare elaborate proprietary selling "models" that they ask representatives to follow during sales calls. The truth is, every sales call takes on a life of its own, and even the best-trained representatives find it impossible follow any model to the letter.

In reality, it's better to think of these selling models as road maps that illustrate the main highways. When your real journey is under way, you'll actually travel down many side roads (hopefully avoiding the dead ends) before you reach your destination.

Skills training requires a lot of practice, a lot of repetition, and a lot of role-playing activities. This type of training is packed with lectures, exercises, and activities. A series of 8-hour days of this intensity can be stressful for a new representative. But it is essential for helping you to absorb and model the selling behaviors that enable physicians to decide to prescribe your company's products. You'll learn more about selling skills and the sales call in Chapters 7 and 8.

Some representatives discover that learning all the clinical and marketplace information is relatively easy and that practicing selling skills is more difficult. Others find that the opposite true–that selling skills and communications skills come easily, but that clinical and market knowledge represents drudgery.

For me, the "academic" portion of my training was relatively easy, perhaps because I was always a good student with good study habits. As far as my interpersonal skills, I (like many people) was terrified of public speaking. During training I was terribly apprehensive about delivering presentations to trainers, managers, or a room full of salespeople. In fact, on one day that I was scheduled to deliver a presentation, I was so nervous that I drank half a bottle of Pepto-Bismol to settle my stomach!

The message here is: It's okay to be nervous. It happens to a lot of us.

About your trainers

As a new hire, you will probably be working under the tutelage of your company's training managers. Generally, these are former representatives who earned promotions after several years of success in the field.

A good trainer understands that anxiety is common among trainees and will ensure that the environment is supportive and non-judgmental. Within a reasonably short period, you'll discover that your stress level diminishes. Repetition, plus positive feedback and constructive critiques fuel your confidence.

As is the case with your DM, the job of the trainer is to make you better. Trainers are your allies who are responsible for teaching and/or testing you on all of the knowledge and skills you will need in the field.

Your trainers will provide you with practical applications for all of the material you have learned regarding disease, treatments, product knowledge, and marketplace understanding.

Trainers will deliver PowerPoint and flipchart presentations, introduce guest speakers, provide self-study assignments, facilitate games and exercises, and quiz you on content. They will introduce you to and coach you in more advanced levels of communications skills such as:

• handling of customer questions and concerns

- listening and questioning skills
- use and interpretation of clinical studies in sales calls

We'll take a closer look at all of these issues later. The point that I want to stress here is that during training you must demonstrate to your trainers' satisfaction a mastery of clinical and marketplace knowledge, as well as the requisite selling and communication skills. Only then will your trainers turn you loose in the field to begin calling on physicians.

As you contemplate that first sales call, remember that your company has invested a lot in your training and has a lot riding on your performance in the field. It's up to you to ensure that this investment pays off.

Physicians don't see your chief executive officer or vice president of sales or chief research scientist. They see you. To the customer, *you* are the corporation.

Tips while training

I've been on both sides in the training environment, and here's my advice to a new hire training for the first time.

- *Ask **lots** of questions during training sessions and breaks (but not after 6 p.m. when your trainer probably wants to vacate the conference room and enjoy informal socializing and dinner with the class).*
- *Find a friend or create a group of colleagues to study and role-play with. Communication is a critical part of the job so start now making new friends and practicing communication skills.*
- *Anticipate—and be receptive to—constructive criticism. Your DM and training managers have seen many people come and go, and they have served in the field themselves. They know what it takes to be successful. They are on your side.*

- *Focus on **one** issue at a time. You accumulate knowledge and skills gradually, item by item. If you receive a weeklong training agenda, focus on what you need to do **today**. That's all.*
- *Take breaks. If you are camped out in a hotel room—or your home office—with piles of books and audiocassettes, recognize fatigue and stress. Complete a workout or go for a walk, run, or swim.*
- *Take risks. Training is the perfect environment for making mistakes. If, for example, you are afraid of speaking in front of a group, take the risk and be the first to volunteer for a role-play. Make your mistakes in front of your colleagues, not in front of doctors.*
- *Resist the temptation to eat. Pharmaceutical companies are exceptionally generous when it comes to providing food when representatives gather at hotels and conference centers for training events. Following a buffet breakfast, it's pastries and fresh fruit in midmorning (stick with the fruit), a huge lunch, cookies and brownies (and maybe more fruit—stay with it) at mid-afternoon, followed by cocktails and a big dinner in the evening. You'll also discover big bowls of candies in front of you all day long. In other words, there's enough food for your group in a day to feed an entire third-world country. A former trainee I knew gained 15 pounds in one month of training—mostly on M&M consumption. I'm not kidding.*
- *Stay positive. A positive outlook is essential in training and throughout your selling career. Training may seem endless and oppressive at times, and you will encounter rejection in the field from time to time. It's all part of the process. There are many texts, videos, and professionals who make a lot of money regarding motivation in a selling career.*

Chapter 5

Getting Organized

I vividly remember the days shortly after I was hired as a pharmaceutical sales representative. I recall the thrill I experienced when I started receiving huge shipping cartons, courtesy of my new employer...one box right after another, day after day, for several days. And this was in *addition* to all the training materials I mentioned in the last chapter.

The cartons were packed with what seemed like tons of colorful binders, marketing literature, special equipment (such as a portable video monitor and a display case), product samples, and giveaway items (coffee mugs, pens, mousepads, clipboards, notepads, etc.).

The thrill wore off pretty quickly. For one thing, I ran out of space to store the stuff. For another, I felt overwhelmed. At least with Book-of-the-Month Club and Columbia House, you can cancel your membership if they keep sending you unwanted merchandise. When you work for a pharmaceutical company, cancellation is not an option. Cancellation is not a good idea anyway because you *need* it all. Unfortunately, building an addition onto your house to accommodate all the materials is not often feasible.

This all goes to say that your company will send you a *lot* of materials. And you will be well served to plan in *advance* as to where you will store it and how you will organize it.

In fact, you will need to organize several aspects of your life—your office, your car, your time, and so on—or the requirements of your new career will rapidly overwhelm you. This chapter provides suggestions that provide a jump-start on the organizational skills required for the job.

Your home office

One of the advantages of being a territory representative is that you work out of your own home. This means that you can customize your office to match your own tastes and preferences. For those of you who can't stand working in a tiny cubicle wedged into a maze-like cavern the size of a football field, pharmaceutical selling is a great career choice.

But you still have to organize your workspace. Here are some suggestions:

Choose a location in your home or apartment where you will not be disturbed. Make sure your office has a door to ensure privacy.

Use a large desk or table as you primary workspace. I say large because there will be times when you'll need to spread out a lot of material for easy access.

Purchase a comfortable chair, or borrow one from another part of your house. (My first desk and chair were ones I used as a high school student. I did not have a lot of room to organize things, and I experienced terrible back pain. Don't make the same mistake.)

Select motivational quotes, photographs, potted or hanging plants, and art objects that create an ambiance to match your personal tastes.

Your company will probably provide you with a laptop computer, a printer, and even a fax machine. Make sure you make space for these items.

Purchase all your office supplies *before* you need them. Items should include pens, pencils, whiteboard, erasable markers, yellow high-lighters, stapler, staple remover, tape and dispenser, printer paper, envelopes, paper punch, ruler, calculator, scissors, rubber-bands, paper clips, and so on. You should also have a supply of corporate letterhead stationery, provided by your company.

Purchase a new or used file cabinet: Use it to organize sales litera-ture, clinical studies, and internal correspondence by product. Label your file folders and keep them in alphabetical order. Other examples of items you'll need to file include sales reports, territory and physician analysis reports, quota worksheets, customer and intra-company cor-respondence, starter-sample reports, performance evaluations, busi-ness plans, hospital and MCO profiles, and so on. *Warning:* Don't become a pack rat. Every six months or so, purge those items that you don't need on a regular basis. Otherwise, you will shortly need to pur-chase another file cabinet.

Remember all of those training materials you were introduced to in the last chapter? You'll need space for them. Keep your training materi-als at hand on office storage shelves or in a bookcase. There's no way you'll remember everything that's covered in all of those binders. You will find yourself referring to certain materials again and again.

Make certain that you have space for standard reference books, too. At a minimum, you'll need a regular dictionary, a medical dictionary, and the current PDR.

Selling materials

Many of those cartons you'll receive contain important materials that will support your sales calls. No automobile in the world has enough space to store them all, and your office probably won't be large enough either. I'll provide some storage suggestions in a moment, but first, let's examine a list of what you'll receive:

Product samples: As you'll learn later, providing product samples to physicians is an important part of selling. If your company supplies you with samples (there are some companies that do not sample) you will need to keep accurate records of their distribution. Record-keeping is essential because the FDA keeps close track of sample use.

Utilize the first-in-first-out ("FIFO") method for sample storage. Organize sample cartons so that you can easily see the drug name, dosage strength, and expiration dates. By using the FIFO method to control your sample inventory, you will help ensure that your samples are never out of date. You will not make friends with the physician's staff if your samples expire two days after you deliver them.

Samples for some medications, most notably injectables and liquid suspensions, may have special storage requirements relating to temperature and humidity. You'll find these requirements listed near the end of the package insert. Your company will almost certainly provide you with special instructions, if they are necessary, in a boldfaced cover letter or fax. Always observe these requirements. They may mean that you cannot leave certain products in your car overnight, or even on a hot day. (You may actually need a picnic cooler in which to store some medications.)

Many representatives stack their samples in their cellars. If you do this, stack your samples off the floor on pallets. Moisture can ruin boxes.

Sales literature: You'll receive reams of sales literature to support your promotion of every product. Items typically include:

Visual aids—These are glossy brochures printed on heavy stock that range in length from a single sheet to 8 or 12 pages.

Clinical studies—Clinical studies (which are usually reprinted from medical journal articles) provide statistical proof of your products' efficacy and safety. You will probably have from one to five studies that you will use in the field *per product.* Organize them carefully so that you can find a desired study on a moment's notice.

"Slim Jims"—These are 8½″ x 3½″, pocket-size brochures or booklets that typically summarize promotional messages along with selected data and conclusions from clinical studies. Occasionally, you'll deal with "Big Jims," which serve the same purpose but measure 8½″ x 11″.

Giveaways: Premiums. Freebies. Handouts. Whatever you want to call them. They are everywhere in pharmaceutical sales. These are the pens, notepads, calendars, clocks, magnets, note-holders, coffee mugs, picture frames, wall posters, and so on that every sales representative provides to physicians and their staffs. Of course, every item has the product's logo printed on it in big bold letters. The idea is that when the doctor sees your product's name, he or she will remember to prescribe the drug the next time a patient shows up with the appropriate diagnosis. You'll receive cartonloads of these items, and you'll need space in which to store them.

Watch out for "giveaway creep"!

Giveaway items are neat. Most of them are functional, and you'll find them useful around your own home. But watch out for "giveaway creep," the term I use to describe the slow and insidious way that marketing items found their way into my household.

I woke up and punched the snooze alarm on a company clock. I showered and dried off with a company towel. I blew my nose with company tissue from a company dispenser.

I opened a refrigerator door adorned with my children's photographs mounted on my company's magnetized frames. I drank coffee from a company mug and consumed bacon and eggs served on a company plate. I patted my face with a company napkin.

When I answered the phone, I took notes with a company pen on a company pad.

Before I left my house, I checked the date on a company calendar, and my second cup of coffee went into a company travel mug.

*I played tennis in a company shirt and quenched my thirst from a company water bottle. I once played tennis against a representative from another company, and we played with his company's **tennis balls**. (They were designed as replicas of a company product, which was dispensed as a round, bright yellow tablet.)*

I played golf in yet another company shirt with company balls, company tees, company repair tool, company towel, and company umbrella.

Before I went to sleep, I marked my place with a company bookmark. AAAAAhhhhhhhhh....!

My message is this...Giveaways are designed for customers and their support staffs. Use these items in the manner for which are intended. Get rid of them appropriately or they may take over your life!

The storage challenge

So where do you store all of these items if you live in an apartment or small home?

If your company allows you to expense a rental storage unit you should do so. When you consider the volume of materials you'll receive, a 10' x 12' storage space might be sufficient

Of course, you will save your company some money and yourself a lot of time if you can find a way to store everything on your own premises. Basements and garages (if the environment is humidity free) are good places to start.

Be careful, however. If boxes start accumulating in the garage, you may force a car out into the driveway, which may not please your housemates, especially on cold winter mornings.

Your detail bag

There's another package that the delivery person will drop off some day. Open the carton and you'll discover a black leather rectangular box with a carry handle. This is your "detail bag." Actually, it's not a "bag" at all, but a customized briefcase. Customized to the point that it looks like an ordinary briefcase injected with growth hormones.

Your detail bag is carried like a briefcase and will hold product samples sufficient for one or two calls, depending upon your degree of generosity on any given day. You'll find space on the other side of the bag to store promotional literature and clinical studies. *Always* keep your detail bag neat and well organized so that you can produce a desired item on a moment's notice.

Detail bags are available in two sizes: regular and petite. The smaller version is designed for female representatives. When in the field, the ideal spot for your detail bag is in the trunk of your car next to all the samples, product literature, and giveaways. This way, you can "reload" each time you return to your vehicle. The company may also provide you with a small hand cart or "dolly" on which to place the bag as well as additional items you need to carry but cannot manage all at once. If you do not receive this dolly it would be a good idea to go to your local office supply store and buy one. It will pay for itself many times over.

Some reps don't like the official pharmaceutical representative black detail bag and select their own oversized briefcase. This is fine as long as you maintain a professional appearance. Don't select one that is too large. You don't want to look like you are on your way to play in a hockey game.

Your car

You'll spend lots of time in your car, so that's the next place to organize. Without careful planning and continuous upkeep, your car will very quickly become an unsightly clutter zone. You'll also have difficulty locating the precise clinical study that you need on a moment's notice, such as when you have a chance encounter with a key physician in a hospital parking lot. It happens to every representative, and physicians rarely have time to wait while you rummage through your trunk looking for the right study.

You have your family and friends to consider, too. You want to avoid the need to engage in a major archeological excavation project every time you have a backseat passenger.

Here are some car-management suggestions that made life easier in my career:

- Cut the tops off the sample boxes in your trunk. Keep samples organized by drug and dosage strength. Have extra boxes on hand for fast-moving products. Try to keep samples out of the seating area where someone could be tempted to steal them or where they will cook on a hot day. (Remember: Don't store them in the car for long periods of time if they are subject to temperature requirements.)

- On the passenger side, keep an open box containing current give-away items. Have extra boxes of popular giveaways in the back seat or trunk.

- Keep all sales literature (sales aids, clinical studies, etc.) in a portable, top-opening hanging-file box. Organize literature by product, and clearly label index tabs.

- Have a good utility knife on hand to open boxes. (Be careful. I've occasionally sliced a hand or finger when I was in a hurry, so I carried a box of Band-aids, too!)

- Keep a box of business cards handy. They tend to disappear very quickly.

- Keep an extra car key in your wallet or purse or in a hideaway place on the exterior of your vehicle. (I am one of the several pharmaceutical representatives who have walked out of a successful call, beaming broadly and full of confidence, only to find that I locked myself out of my car.)

- Buy a safety kit at a local Wal-Mart. You should always have flares, jumper cables, a flashlight, and a blanket…just in case.
- Store an umbrella in the backseat or trunk. Personal appearance counts. You want to look your absolute best, even when you have to cross a parking lot in a tropical downpour.
- Keep accurate, up-to-date maps covering all your territory. (Some companies now provide representatives with electronic mapping/homing devices. Key in the address of a physician's office, and—presto!—the route appears in front of you.)

While I'm on the subject of cars, here are some other suggestions to observe while traveling:

- Maintain a supply of spare change for tolls and parking.
- Keep sunglasses in the car.
- Always wear your seatbelt.
- Don't park directly in front of physician offices. Those spots are for patients.
- Keep your laptop computer covered or under the front seat when you are not using it.
- Don't use your cell phone or look at your computer when driving. (You're supposed to be visiting doctors. Having a doctor visit you while you are in a hospital room following an auto accident is a clever tactic, but it probably won't help you make your sales goals.)
- Record your sample transactions after every call. Accurate sample records are critically important. Don't procrastinate.

Another very useful item for your vehicle is a trunk protector. This is a mat that lines the bottom of your trunk and folds out over your bumper when you are rummaging through everything. It helps protect your clothes from getting soiled when coming in contact with the back of the vehicle.

Your car is your sanctuary

In my days in the field, my car was my sanctuary. I established a comfort zone there, and there were certain occasions when I dreaded stepping outside. It may have been because of pouring rain, driving snow, frigid cold, or intense heat and humidity. Or maybe I was just having a bad day (everyone does) or was apprehensive about an imminent meeting with a particularly difficult customer.

When that happened, I'd always pause for a moment to ponder all the more satisfying days I've experienced as well. I considered that, compared to other places I might be in the business world, on balance, this was the best place for me to be. I was free to manage my own time in the pursuit of my professional responsibilities.

Perhaps you have had a job where you sat in a tiny cubicle in an impersonal office building breathing recycled air and listening to white noise all day. Chances are, you didn't even have a window. And chances are, someone else micromanaged every minute of your day.

As a sales representative, you can drive down almost any street or parkway in your territory and enjoy the scenery, or perhaps the hustle and bustle of a major metropolitan area. It's a great life, and many people would kill for a job with so much freedom. Receptionists and office staff where you make your sales calls will be jealous of you...you'll see.

Organizing your time

We've talked about organizing materials and space. Let's move on to another critical area that demands the utmost in organizing skills—your time.

The freedom associated with being a territory representative involves responsibility and a lot of very hard work. You must map out every week almost to the hour. You must prepare a plan for every call you plan to make. You must also be prepared for the calls you *don't* plan to make, such as chance encounters with doctors in hallways, elevators, and parking lots.

The more organized you are about this, the easier it will be to accomplish your goals, which are to:

Visit and talk with as many physicians as possible in a prioritized manner. ("Prioritized" means seeing your best prospects—the "high prescribers" and most influential physicians—first.)

Address all of the other responsibilities required to support your selling activities. These responsibilities include traveling to and from your storage unit (to retrieve and organize materials); ordering and picking up (or arranging for delivery) of an office lunch for a valued customer; meeting with your DM or other members of the sales team; filling out reports; attending training sessions; it never ends.

Obviously, if you are just making calls all the time and not attending to your other responsibilities, your inattentiveness to your support chores will catch up with you. Chaos will follow.

Conversely, if you become obsessed with planning and organizing, you won't have time to make your call quotas, and productivity will suffer.

I've seen it work both ways among my colleagues. You have to strike the proper balance. You must prioritize your selling *and* administrative responsibilities, and you must manage your time in a manner that works for you.

In summary, plan your work, and work your plan.

Time management tips

You'll quickly discover that the position of pharmaceutical sales representative can be a 24-hour, 7-day-a-week job—but only if you allow that to happen. This is because of countless administrative and support tasks that come with the job of actually selling.

Here are some suggestions that can help you address your time management challenges:

Make a list. Make a list of all the administrative items you need to address. The list will include expense reports, writing the article for the company newsletter, calling your DM, filing, creating invitations for a guest speaker, completing a weekly call report, taking your suits to the cleaners, re-organizing your storage unit, etc.

Then, *prioritize* your list by identifying:

- Items that absolutely need to get done *today* because their completion is critical to the success of your territory.
- Items that must be done *this week* in order for you to stay up-to-date and organized.
- Items that are low-priority that can be done in your *spare time* (what little you'll have).

Obviously, you need to take care of the #1 items first, then proceed to the #2's and #3's If you are like me, you have a tendency—or compulsion—to take care of the #3 items first. How come? Because it always takes less effort to deal with the low-hanging fruit. Surfing the web, reading *Pharm Rep* magazine, or chatting with a colleague about "no-see" doctors is much easier than planning a dinner program for 20 nurse practitioners or writing a report on yesterday's sales presentation at the regional health fair.

Check off items on the list as you complete them. This provides you with a feeling of accomplishment, and you can track your progress.

Manage your communications. Set up a speed dial directory so that you can call your DM and key customers without having to consult a card file or phone directory. When in your office, screen your incoming calls. Obviously, pick up the phone if your DM is on the line (trust me, there will be occasions when you won't want to, but do it anyway). Return calls later if it's a friend inquiring about Saturday's golf match or this week's investment club meeting.

Manage your correspondence and other documentation. This includes "snail mail," e-mail, and faxes. Regardless of the media, read important, need-to-know business correspondence immediately. Save the nice-to-know material for later. Trash the junk mail right away. For outgoing correspondence, store frequently used addresses in your computer, and create preprinted labels for addresses that you use routinely.

Keep a generous supply of stationery and stamps on hand at all times. *Always* proofread any correspondence generated in your word processor—letters, faxes, e-mails, reports, customer invitations, etc. Check for content and grammatical accuracy as well as spelling. If English is not your strong suit, find a colleague who's willing to check your work on important documents.

Save computer work frequently and back up to disk or text often. Transmit copies of important work to appropriate directories in your company's documentation system for safe storage. (I can't tell you how often I have worked hours on critical documents and lost them without appropriate backups.)

Routinely purge your system of outdated files to make room for newly created documents.

Use an organized time-management or calendaring system. I highly recommend that you use an organized electronic time-management or calendaring system. Very often your desktop or laptop computer will have a system built into it.

I like programs that can print out appointment schedules that can be referred to in the field. I have found that the Franklin-Covey system works best for me. It's especially helpful because it allows you to schedule your professional life while incorporating family and personal activities that are also essential for your well-being. This provides a balanced approach that helps contribute to a desirable lifestyle. This system is available in text and in software that works nicely in a Palm-Pilot for those of you who are comfortable with hand-held software.

Here are a few additional tips on time management for the pharmaceutical sales rep:

- Prioritize *all* of your daily activities. Create a *weekly* list Sunday night or early Monday morning, well ahead of the time when you begin your sales call activity. Plan on calling on the high-volume cities and towns first. Next, call on the high-prescribing physicians, according to your company's physician profiling data. (Data is usually provided in the form of computer printouts provided by a pharmacy benefit manager or prescription data management company and includes prescribing volume by therapeutic category and, in some cases, individual brands.)
- Then, plan each *day* ahead of time, before you leave your office. Cluster your calls by geographic area so you don't have to backtrack during the day.
- Check your e-mail *at least* twice a day, morning and evening. Prioritize your responses as suggested earlier.
- Check your voice mail *no more* than three times a day. Voice mail is a killer for a pharmaceutical representative. It's very easy to become addicted to that cell phone. When you do receive a voice mail, reply immediately *only* if your response is critical to the success of your territory or district *today*.
- Fill out all call-activity and sample reports *after each call*. Do not slip into the very bad habit of waiting until the end of the day (or week or, heaven forbid…the month) to do this. The first reason for this is simple: When recording this information immediately, you will remember what you and the doctor discussed with much more clarity and accuracy; and you will recall precisely the volume of samples you left behind. These factors will help ensure that your next call is successful. The second reason is that, when you accomplish these tasks in the field, you will spend less time in your office at home and more time with your family, friends, and personal activities.

- Recognize your procrastination habits and correct them. For example, if you exhibit the tendency to move on to the next call before recording information from the preceding one, you might place a photograph of your children on your dashboard. This will remind you that time at home is better spent with them than in your office trying to recall the details of your visit with Dr. Smith.

If you are involved in teamwork activities, it's okay to volunteer for extra work, but be careful. Make certain that your colleagues are sharing the workload. Delegate when appropriate.

When waiting to see a physician, read your company literature, work on your planner, or mentally rehearse your presentation. It might be tempting to browse through *People* or *Sports Illustrated*. Don't do it. (Keep in mind that the periodicals are probably at least a year old anyway.)

Avoid taking on tasks that take you away from your primary mission. If a colleague in an adjacent territory asks for assistance at a hospital display, it may be necessary to politely turn the person down, citing responsibilities in your own territory. I'm a big believer in teamwork whenever it contributes to personal productivity. Use common sense.

Talking with the competition—yes or no?

I would venture to guess that on nearly a third of your sales calls, you will encounter at least one representative from another pharmaceutical firm—either in the parking lot, a hallway, or waiting area.

This individual may or may not be in direct competition with you. For example, if you are selling a blood pressure drug, the other representative might be promoting a similar drug head-to-head. Then again, he or she may be selling an influenza vaccine or an antidepressant, and the competition is only for the physician's time.

Whatever the scenario, most competitive representatives will become familiar faces to you over time. Some will even become your friends.

Just remember this: You are in the field to promote your company's products, not to socialize with competitive representatives. If you happen to stop and chat with another pharmaceutical representative, keep your conversation brief. It's easy to get into a 20- to 30-minute conversation only to notice that the doctor you wanted to see is leaving the office to go to the hospital—or play golf. (I confess that I "lost" doctors in this manner on several occasions.)

I once had a senior manager whom absolutely forbade talking to the competition altogether. While I was somewhat sympathetic to his reasoning, I have to tell you that you will meet some very nice people on competitive sales forces. And if you are not direct competitors, you may even trade tips regarding a particular physician's "hot buttons."

I know of one representative rep who met his future wife while she was working the same territory for another company.

If you do fraternize, be careful about what you say regarding your company and its products. Much information in this industry is confidential. Don't leak any secrets that could harm your company.

Some advice about work habits

Occasionally, you'll find yourself in a doctor's office at 4:30 in the afternoon and someone on staff will say, "What are you doing here? I thought all you reps quit by 3:00."

The reason they say this is because they do tend to see fewer reps toward the end of the day. The fact is that there are a few representatives out there with bad habits. After a few months in the field, you will probably become acquainted with reps who limit their calling hours from 9:00 a.m. to 3:00 p.m. or 10:00 a.m. to 4:00 p.m. A few of these representatives might not even go out when it rains or snows—they might hang out all day in a hospital to avoid the elements.

Don't develop these types of behaviors. It's easy to fall into that trap, but the fact is, if you are creative in varying your selling hours, you'll become more productive, see a higher number of different physicians, and have more fun.

Remember, no one is looking over your shoulder day in and day out telling you where to go, whom to see, or what time to make your calls. You are free to manage your time as you see fit, consistent, of course, with your professional obligation to achieve your sales objectives.

I want to emphasize once more that with freedom comes responsibility and accountability. There are many key attributes shared by top-performing pharmaceutical representatives, including clinical knowledge, awareness of the marketplace, and first-rate communication skills. Another is the willingness to work hard—at times, very hard.

As I said earlier, many representatives are exceptionally talented regarding clinical knowledge, market awareness, and communication skills. These attributes help create a solid foundation for success. But it is those reps who put in a full day, every day, every week, month after month who will reap the cash bonuses that usually come with superior performance. These representatives know the value of "sweat equity" and act accordingly. They are out the door at 8:00 and roll back into the driveway at 6:00 every day.

Truly astute representatives know that bad-weather days (I don't mean when conditions are hazardous or life-threatening) represent some of the best opportunities to see physicians. After all, think of the number of patients (especially elderly patients) who are reluctant to venture out on these days and cancel their appointments. A perfect time to call on doctors!

At the end of the day, always make that last, extra call on your way home. You'll be surprised at how many times this kind of effort pays off. Remember, in golf the difference between the winner of the tournament and the runner-up is often just one stroke, which might be the result of one misaligned putt that missed the hole by a half-inch or less. A pharmaceutical sale can be made or missed in much the same manner.

Very often, at district meetings my manager would display charts and graphs showing the measurable work-activity behaviors of all the representatives in the district. Without exception, representatives who received awards and recognition were those who distributed most samples, made the most calls, delivered the highest number of multiple product presentations, executed a high number physician teleconference calls, and sponsored the greatest number of special programs. Invariably, these individuals received the quickest promotions. (That is, of course, if they wanted to be promoted. Some representatives prefer the freedom that comes with the "territory," and they choose to stay in the field for many years).

Here's a key point: When you start a new position with a pharmaceutical company, you must definitely put in a great deal of time learning the ropes. You have a lot to learn and study, and you have a whole territory of physicians to become familiar with. You must also learn all of your company's policies and procedures. This all takes a lot of time. As the months and years roll by, you become more adept at time management. You'll still put in a full day's work, but after a while your nights and weekends come back to you, as will your family and your friends.

The bottom line is this: The greater the number of minutes that you spend in front of doctors generally corresponds directly to the number of prescriptions for your products. Don't forget however that you have to earn those minutes.

You'll learn how to make the most of those minutes in subsequent chapters. First, you must get to know your customers.

Chapter 6

Meet Your Customers

The primary customer for the pharmaceutical sales representative has always been and probably always will be the physician. Accordingly, you will probably spend most of your time in the field calling on doctors.

Today, however, many other healthcare professionals influence prescribing and, in many locales, it is important for you to know them all. They include everyone from managed care administrators and pharmacists to office nurses and business managers.

While these individuals do not *prescribe* drugs for patients, they often have the clout to determine which drugs are available to physicians and the circumstances in which certain drugs can be used. Certain personnel, especially nurses, can wield considerable influence in physician offices and hospitals. It will be important for you to make these acquaintances in your day-to-day selling.

I will introduce you to some of these other individuals later in this chapter. I'll focus on physicians first.

There are two broad categories of physicians whom you'll call on: primary care physicians and specialists.

Primary care physicians (PCPs)

Primary care physicians (PCPs) represent the first line of care for patients and include:

- general and family practitioners
- internists
- pediatricians

General and family practitioners. General and family practice is actually a broad-based medical specialty. General and family practitioners (GP/FPs) treat patients of all ages for a variety of disorders—everything from the common cold and minor sprains to the flu, bacterial infections, and uncomplicated chronic diseases such as asthma, hypertension (high blood pressure), diabetes, and emphysema. Consequently, GP/FPs must have knowledge of internal medicine, pediatrics, obstetrics, gynecology, surgery, psychiatry, and preventive medicine.

Patients usually select GPs or FPs as their personal physicians. You almost certainly have one yourself, so you probably already have a reasonably good idea of how these physicians diagnose and treat you when you are not feeling well or have a medical problem.

Internists. Internists (IMs) are generalists who focus on the diagnosis and treatment of diseases affecting the internal organs (the heart, kidneys, gastrointestinal tract, etc.). Because IMs are familiar with a variety of organ systems, many patients use internists as PCPs.

Generally, about half of an IM's patients are 60 years old or older. Because older patients tend to suffer from a higher number of chronic conditions than the rest of the population, they tend to require a higher volume of prescription drugs. Therefore, internists make excellent targets for sales calls.

Pediatricians. Pediatricians are generalists who specialize in the treatment of children, from birth to age 15 or 18. Like other PCPs, pediatricians treat a wide variety of disorders. Obviously, pediatricians are most interested in pharmaceutical products with pediatric applications, especially antibiotics, vaccines, and nutritional supplements.

PCPs and pharmaceutical selling

Generally speaking, most newly-hired pharmaceutical representatives promote their products almost exclusively to PCPs. There are several reasons for this. For one thing, PCPs represent the first line of care in the healthcare system, so they see the highest number of patients and prescribe a high volume of drugs. For another, PCPs also diagnose and treat the common diseases and conditions for which the most popular prescription medications are designed to treat. These include:

- anxiety and depression
- arthritis
- asthma and allergies
- bacterial infections
- cold and flu
- diabetes
- gastrointestinal disorders
- high blood pressure
- high cholesterol
- pain
- sexually transmitted diseases

Another reason that new hires typically call on PCPs is because a new representative's level of knowledge (following new-hire training) generally matches the requirements associated with promoting to PCPs. Promoting to specialists usually demands a higher level of scientific knowledge that comes with experience in the field or advanced training by your company.

Whether or not a company's new hires call exclusively on PCPs relates directly to the structure of the sales force and the nature of the product. A company that sells a blood pressure drug may train all of its territory representatives to call on PCPs and cardiologists, while another company that sells a similar product may manage two separate sales forces—one for PCPs and one for cardiologists—both of which sell the same drug to their respective target audiences.

Of course, if a company specializes in high-level ophthalmalogical products, then all representatives for that company—rookies and veterans alike—will call exclusively on ophthalmologists, and representatives will be trained accordingly.

Specialists

PCPs provide primary care for their patients and often help patients manage early-stage chronic diseases (such as asthma or cardiovascular disease.). PCPs generally refer patients to specialists when:

- chronic disease progresses to the point where it requires the attention of an expert in that disease
- chronic disease becomes complicated by another disease (e.g., a diabetic patient is diagnosed with heart disease)[*]
- the PCP seeks confirmation of a diagnosis in a specialist's field of expertise (In many situations, after confirmation, the specialist refers the patient back to the PCP for primary care and continues consulting with the PCP during the course of treatment.)
- a patient requires surgery
- the PCP is unable or not qualified to make a definitive diagnosis (for example, when a patient presents with a tumor, the PCP would refer the patient to an oncologist; with a vision problem,

---

[*]The presence of two or more diseases in an individual at the same time is referred to as "comorbidity," a term that you will encounter frequently during your pharmaceutical sales career.

to an ophthalmologist; with a foot problem, to a podiatrist; and so on)

Specialists possess advanced degrees in their fields of expertise. A specialist's professional focus is far narrower than that of a PCPs, but his or her level of knowledge regarding the specialty is much higher. In other words, you can anticipate that a specialist's knowledge of anatomy, physiology, pathophysiology,** and pharmacology regarding his or her specialty is highly advanced.

Does this mean that when you call on a specialist that your knowledge of these issues must be highly advanced as well?

Yes, at least relative to the knowledge you must possess when you call on PCPs all the time. For example, both PCPs and cardiologists prescribe blood pressure drugs. A PCP might simply be interested in the fact that a product works (it lowers blood pressure) and is safe (side effects are minimal). On the other hand, a cardiologist who is considering the same drug might want to know about its pharmacokinetic profile (what happens to the drug over time as it passes through the body) and its suitability for patients who suffer from chronic renal failure, diabetes, or heart failure,

That's just a general rule. Certain PCPs will demand some fairly sophisticated data about your products, while some specialists will prescribe it with hardly a glance at your supportive documentation.

Still, if you promote exclusively to specialists, assume that your knowledge of a particular branch of medicine must be far more advanced than it would be if you were selling exclusively to PCPs. Don't worry, though, your company will provide appropriate training—and if you get in over your head occasionally (it has happened to me), you always have a bail-out option (See box).

**Pathophysiology refers to functional changes in the body that accompany a disease.

When you don't have the answer...

What if a doctor says something like...

"Your product sounds very beneficial. But tell me, in Phase III trials, what were the endogenous baseline serum erythropoietin levels among patients who were receiving concomitant non-cisplatin-containing chemotherapy?"

...and you have no clue what she is talking about. (Trust me, from time to time you'll encounter physicians who press your buttons with questions just like this one.)

If you don't have the answer, admit it, and tell the doctor you will get back to her with a response. After the sales call, get in touch with your company's Medical Department (every company has one, usually accessible by e-mail), ask the same question to the department representative, and he or she will get back to the physician with the response (with a copy to you).

There will be some cases in which it will be appropriate to advise the physician to directly access the medical department with a toll free number. You will learn about these situations in your training.

Common physician specialties and subspecialties include:
- *Allergist.* Treats patients with allergic reactions, as well as patients with asthma.
- *Anesthesiologist.* Administers anesthetics (agents that cause a loss of sensation).
- *Cardiologist.* Addresses diseases of the heart and circulatory system. May subspecialize in cardiovascular surgery.
- *Dermatologist.* Diagnoses and treats skin disorders.
- *Emergency medicine (EM) specialist.* Addresses medical emergencies such as heart attacks and trauma.

- *Endocrinologist.* Deals with hormonal disorders—diabetes is the most common.
- *Gastroneterologist.* Treats disorders of the esophagus, stomach, and intestines.
- *General surgeon.* Surgically treats disorders and injuries, usually involving the abdomen, the hormone system, and circulation.
- *Gerontologist.* Specializes in medical problems associated with aging.
- *Hematologist.* Treats disorders of the blood.
- *Immunologist.* Addresses disorders of the body's immune system (such as HIV/AIDs).
- *Nephrologist.* Focuses on the diagnosis and treatment of kidney disorders.
- *Neurologist.* Deals with disorders of the nervous system.
- *Neurosurgeon.* Practices surgery specific to the brain and nervous system.
- *Obstetrician/gynecologist (OB/GYN).* Is concerned with pregnancy, labor, delivery, postnatal care, and women's reproductive health. (Often a PCP for women.)
- *Oncologist.* Addresses problems associated with malignant (life-threatening) tumors.
- *Opthalmologist.* Diagnoses and treats eye and vision disorders and diseases.
- *Orthopedist.* Diagnoses and corrects problems related to bones and associated structures, often surgically.
- *Osteopath.* Treats patients by restoring the physical and physiological integrity of the body through manipulation, surgery, and medication.
- *Otolaryngologist.* Deals with disorders of the ear, nose, and upper respiratory tract. Also called an "ear, nose, and throat specialist," or ENT.
- *Pathologist.* Focuses on the laboratory study and diagnosis of diseases, their origins, developments, and consequences.
- *Psychiatrist.* Diagnoses and treats mental and emotional disorders.

- *Pulmonologist.* Treats patients with diseases and disorders of the lungs.
- *Radiologist.* Uses x-ray technology to assist other physician in the diagnosis and treatment of disease.
- *Rheumatologist.* Focuses on joint and tissue diseases, most notably rheumatoid arthritis.
- *Urologist.* Treats diseases and disorders of the male urinary and genital tracts.

PCPs vs. specialists: What's the difference when selling?

I have found that, although selling to specialists requires far more clinical knowledge than selling to PCPs, specialist calls were more fun. Somehow, I seemed to develop stronger relationships with my specialists, and many other representatives report the same experience.

This is probably because many specialists tend to be "opinion leaders" relating to your product. This means that they may have assisted your company as a clinical study investigator, grand rounds speaker, or formulary advocate.

Though the relationship is typically deeper, so are the expectations of your specialist customers. Very often, they will want you to serve as an advocate for them within your company for new clinical trials or research funding for their institution (in the form of unrestricted educational grants). Specialists may also look to you to help "expand their practices" by mentioning them as referral sources when you call on PCPs.

Specialists typically have more "bells and whistles" at their disposal and I think more camaraderie than their PCP counterparts. These bells and whistles depend upon the specialty. For example, cardiologists are associated with catheterization laboratories, or "cath labs." After you develop a relationship with a cardiologist, he or she may allow you in the lab to observe procedures.

On many instances I would, for example, walk into a prominent Boston hospital looking for a few key CVD customer physicians. I was often told they were in the lab. All I had to do was put on "the lead," enter the lab, and observe cardiac catheterization procedures. I enjoyed watching these procedures and hanging out with physicians in the lab. My experience reminded me of the movie "M*A*S*H" because of the camaraderie among the staff. Somehow, they managed a running commentary with me while simultaneously joking with the nurses or lamenting the inevitable collapse of the Boston Red Sox.

One of the hospitals on my call schedule was exceptionally prestigious and located in downtown Boston. When you tell someone who also has worked in Boston that you have "walked the pike" (the main corridor of this institution), they tend to give you a bit more respect.

This is for two reasons. First, Boston has a reputation for having some of the best clinical and research hospitals in the country. It was a great experience for me being around cutting edge medicine and clinical trials before their results were published in prestigious journals.

Second, and more importantly from a professional perspective, the hospital is also home to some of the most "Ivory Towered" physicians in the world. Securing any degree of success in this institution demanded that I eat a great deal of humble pie in order to secure time with and earn the respect of physicians.

Fun in "The Ivory Tower"

Fortunately, I was able to gain an occasional audience with some otherwise "no-see" physicians at this hospital. One of these was a leading authority on kidney disease and the chief of the nephrology department. He seemed to enjoy playing games of academic cat- and-mouse with me and my selling partner.

He would allow us in to his office suite (high up in the Ivory Tower, of course) and say to us, "Well boys what have you got for me today?"

One day, I replied, "Doctor, your colleague downstairs, the director of your dialysis department, feels very strongly that [drug name] is an exceptionally effective treatment for hypertension and is also friendly on kidney function as well."

The doctor shook his head and responded. "That guy's a knuckle-head! Let me tell you what he *doesn't* know about kidney function." Then he would not only proceed to completely tear down the dialysis guy, he would take amusement in dissecting any journal article that we dared to present.

Still, as much as he was a high-minded, Ivory Tower icon who held his colleagues in absolute fear, he actually enjoyed our visits. In the end he was always helpful to steer us to the clinicians who wrote the most prescriptions and would allow them to make up their own minds regarding their prescription selections.

This doctor was very skilled at securing financial support for his department. For instance, he would say something like, "Boys, we need to bring in a grand rounds speaker next month. Can you help me out?"

I would say, "Gee, Doctor, we have only so much money left in our budget."

He would reply, "Good. Let's spend it!"

Off to see the "Wizard"

Here's another anecdote regarding my experience with a specialist...

Do you recall in *The Wizard of Oz* when Dorothy and the others earned an audience with the Wizard? Remember how the lion was so scared he couldn't even stand up?

Well, after two years of attempts, I finally earned the opportunity to meet with the Chief of Medicine at this most august institution. He was the author of numerous definitive medical textbooks, and principal investigator in many landmark cardiovascular trials.

I believe the reason I got to see him was because he was leading the development of a new healthcare organization in the area. I knew that he must be in need of some type of support of this huge project. My district manager and I asked his secretary to let him know that we were interested in learning about the new organization's objectives and needs and that we would like to assist in any way we could. The gates opened.

For many months, I had dubbed this physician "The Wizard of Oz," and I felt exactly like the cowardly lion going in. He actually turned out to be very a kind and gentle man. After we discussed the new organization I asked if he was interested in hearing about some new clinical information about our company's product. He agreed and after I delivered my presentation, he simply said, "Oh yes, I know all about it. Thank you for visiting." A proverbial pat on the head! He had actually been involved in the development and clinical assessment of the principal molecule of my product.

Overall, I've met and worked with specialists from many fields, including endocrinology, cardiology, allergy/immunology, psychiatry, rheumatology, nephrology, and so on. Each time I ventured into a new area of specialty, I was intimidated much as I was when I walked into a hospital for the first time. Eventually, I learned that although specialists *really* expect you to know your stuff, they are fun to be around, enjoy discussing challenging clinical subjects with you, and like to share their knowledge with interested listeners (which, as you will see in the next chapter, you must become).

The real big difference when selling to a specialist is to know your clinical studies cold so that you can maintain high-level discussions with the doctors and locate key data on a moment's notice. (You will learn more about clinical studies in Chapter 9.)

My bottom-line advice on specialists is this: Sell to them just as you would to PCPs, but anticipate the need to crank it up a notch or two in terms of the clinical details regarding your product.

Physician group practices

Very few physicians work in individual private practices these days. The economics of solo practice rarely makes it worthwhile. Therefore, most physicians form or enter group practices with other physicians.

Group practices can be as small as two or three doctors that share the same specialty. Other group practices can feature a hundred or more physicians at multiple locations covering primary care and most of the major specialties and subspecialties. Obviously, the advantage of visiting a group practice is that you may have the opportunity to score several "hits" while at a single stop.

I recommend developing a strong relationship with one or two physicians at a practice whom you can visit regularly. Then use those visits to make occasional contact with other physicians at the practice. Scheduling group presentations at some practices may be appropriate from time to time. I'll talk about group selling later.

Hospitals

Some of you will spend a lot of time promoting your products in hospitals. A few of you may even spend *all* of your time selling in hospitals. Hospital selling is much different than office selling. For one thing, you'll spend a lot less time in your car. As noted in Chapter 4, if you sell to a cluster of downtown hospitals in a large city, you can park your car in a garage all day long while you make all your calls.

Selling strategies in hospitals vary according to the styles of individual representatives and the preferences of physicians. Some representatives rarely schedule appointments with hospital-based physicians but simply "work" the hospital on most days, interacting with physicians in offices, corridors, lounges, elevators, the cafeteria, surgical suites—even the emergency room.

Although this sounds like a random activity, it should not be. Each time you enter a hospital you should have the names of at least *six* "must see" physicians on your call list—and have an objective for each call.

Of course, you need to be certain that these top docs are in the hospital on the day that you visit. Some doctors are in the hospital only on certain days of the week, spending the rest of their time teaching or in private practice. If possible, see all the physicians on your list. Then spend the rest of the time with spontaneous interactions with other physicians, nurses, residents, and pharmacists—or performing the special selling activities described below.

When possible, schedule appointments with key physicians (e.g., department heads) in their hospital offices, then use those opportunities to get referrals to other physicians.

Selling in a hospital? Be creative!

Because hospitals are staffed by physicians 24 hours a day, savvy representatives have the opportunity to become creative in securing face time with doctors. I know of one representative who routinely showed up in the ER at 10:00 p.m. or so with pizzas and soft drinks for the ER staff. Why not? Things are usually slow at that time (at least on weeknights), and physicians will take the time to talk with you.

Another representative I knew routinely visited surgical suites at six o'clock in the morning with coffee, bagels, and donuts—just about the time physicians, residents, and support staff start their days, but before patients require attention.

First time in a hospital?

Here are some suggestions when you work a hospital for the first time:

- Visit the hospital pharmacy first and obtain a copy of their guidelines for sales representatives. (You may be required to sign in, state the purpose of your visit, and obtain an ID badge)
- Introduce yourself to the chief of pharmacy, present your business card, identify the products you plan to promote, and check to see that the pharmacy has copies of current product literature and relevant clinical studies.
- Locate the different medical departments that you plan to visit.
- Visit the departments that are appropriate for your product, and schedule appointments with the chiefs of those departments. Ask about special department-level policies for sales representatives.
- Visit the outpatient clinic and ask about access to physicians at the clinic.
- Schedule appointments and lunches with as many physicians as possible.
- Develop relationships with office staff, especially nurses. (Nurses administer most medications in the hospital and often know more than physicians about efficacy and side effects).
- Be prepared at all times. You never know when you'll encounter a targeted physician in a hospital—in a corridor, an elevator, the cafeteria, or the parking lot.

As I noted earlier, hospitals can intimidate an uninitiated representative, but if you follow the suggestions outlined here, you'll quickly advance into a comfort zone that will help you earn substantial rewards.

One aspect of hospital work that I love most is its sheer unpredictability. One minute you can be chatting with a first-year resident. The next minute you can be discussing a journal article with one of the most influential endocrinologists in the country. You never know.

Keep in mind that each hospital has its own rules and has its own "personality." You may visit huge urban hospitals that cover a city block or more, or small city hospitals where virtually everyone knows you on a first-name basis.

Special hospital selling activities

Hospital representatives rarely get locked into a daily routine because there are so many channels through which you can approach your targeted customers. In addition to presenting to physicians in their hospital offices (or wherever else in the hospital you can find them), you will find opportunities to:

- set up and sell at hospital displays
- deliver presentations to groups of physicians, pharmacy personnel, and nursing staff
- sponsor inservice training and continuing medical education (CME) programs for physicians, pharmacy personnel, and nursing staff
- attend grand rounds (which are education programs for physicians, medical students and other staff), interacting with key players before and after
- sponsor outside experts to speak at a grand rounds session that relates to your product's indications, and at staff meetings, department meetings, and luncheons
- staff your company's booth at national and regional hospital conferences

Providing food at hospital events is an accepted part of your job, and you will have many opportunities to keep your customers happy in that regard (and they *will* remember the representatives who provide the most scrumptious offerings).

All of these selling channels require different selling skills and protocols for representatives. Your company will provide appropriate training through your training department, DM, or colleagues in the field.

Physicians in training

In the hospital setting—especially in teaching hospitals—you will encounter physicians-in-training on an almost daily basis. It's important to know these customers because they represent your future business. You will get to know these individuals better if you understand how physicians are trained.

A physician's education lasts from eight to fourteen years. The first step is a four-year undergraduate degree, wither a Bachelor of Science (BS) or Bachelor of Arts (BA), usually in a "pre-med" curriculum that emphasizes biomedical science.

Next comes medical school, a four-year program that produces a Doctor of Medicine (MD) degree. Generally, the first two years of medical school lay the theoretical foundation for clinical training, which occurs in the third and fourth years. During clinical training, aspiring physicians have their first opportunities to treat patients, under the supervision of experienced MDs.

During their third year, medical students complete six-week "rotations" in psychiatry, OB/GYN, and pediatrics, as well as twelve-week rotations in internal medicine and general surgery. Medical students then select rotations (called "elective clerkships") in their fourth year of medical school.

After graduating from medical school, MDs must pass national examinations to become licensed in the state(s) in which they wish to practice...but their schooling is not done. As the next step, MDs must complete a one-year internship in internal medicine (called "PGY-1," for "Postgraduate Year One").

Following their internships, many physicians enter general practice as a GP/FP, IM, or pediatrician. However, most physicians complete a hospital residency, a period of clinical training in a chosen specialty. Residency programs vary in length, depending on the specialty selected. Residencies can last up to three to five years or even longer. If you sell in hospitals, it's important to know that residents have prescribing privileges (see box).

There's yet another stop on the long path of medical education—a fellowship. Many physicians choose to pursue advanced study or research as fellows. Fellowships usually last two years or longer. After completing fellowships, physicians can apply to appropriate subspecialty boards for certification.

As mentioned above, you'll have many opportunities in the hospital to provide food for your customers, and residents are often the most appreciative recipients of your largesse. You will have opportunities to provide food for residents at:

- M & M clubs: No, you do not serve chocolate candies here. In fact, these events are nowhere near as sweet as they sound. The M & M, in this case, stands for morbidity and mortality, and it's a regular meeting at which residents complete a case study review of admitted patients.
- Journal clubs: Residents gather once a week or once a month to discuss recently published clinical studies. If a study relates to your product, plan on being there to answer questions.
- Noon reports: These are luncheon meetings at which the hospital's chief-resident reviews current events of note. A physician from the faculty usually follows with a half-hour lecture.

Make friends with residents!

If you sell in a teaching hospital, keep in mind that dozens of residents may rotate through the hospital every year and that most prescriptions in teaching hospitals originate with residents.

Residents are generally young, friendly, and eager to learn about available products and services. They also tend to be more approachable than established physicians. They are more likely to attend your continuing medical education (CME) programs and are often willing to utilize newer drug treatments.

Many residents develop lifelong product preferences and prescribing habits during their residencies, so this is an excellent time to "capture" them with your promotional messages, product literature, and journal articles.

*The **chief resident** could be your most influential contact among residents. This individual is usually a third-year resident who has been selected by the chief of his or her chosen specialty on the basis of ability. The chief resident performs both an administrative and educational function, and other residents look to the chief resident for guidance regarding therapeutic decisions.*

When I first met a physician who was new to my territory he told me that he always made it a point to see representatives from my company because of how well he was treated by my company's representative when he was in residency. That's teamwork over time!

Billiards on Thursday

Work with residents can be lots of fun. Residents are typically under enormous pressure and appreciate opportunities to participate in outside activities.

At one time in my selling career, I had an excellent relationship with the residents at a very prestigious hospital . Unfortunately, the program tightly restricted residents' interactions with non-healthcare professionals in the hospital.

It was interesting to note, however, that the majority of the residents strongly wanted these interactions because the pharmaceutical industry often provides valuable educational resources that most resident programs cannot afford.

Along with a colleague, I decided to create a forum in which residents could take advantage of these resources in a relaxed, after-hours setting. Accordingly, on the third Thursday of every month, we offered an open invitation for the residents to attend a local restaurant to play billiards, enjoy a buffet of cold cuts, and receive some very valuable professional information. Part way through the evening, we stopped all activities, gathered participants around a table, and distributed clinical information. (Yes, we really *did* do the education part.) Typically we showed slides related to clinical trials and distributed reprints for discussion.

The program was a remarkable success. The residents had fun, socialized, and ate heartily—all activities that they rarely had time or money for. Of course, they also obtained education and product information that was professionally beneficial.

Incidentally, this type of activity is completely proper under terms of Food and Drug Administration drug promotion guidelines because it is fair-balanced and there is no return favor or any other type of expectation attached to the program. To avoid potential problems, *always* check with your manager before implementing a program of this nature (e.g., be sure that your invitations indicate that there will be a medical education portion to the program).

Other "targets" for pharmaceutical sales

Physician offices and hospitals are the principal sites where most of your selling activities will take place. However, there are many other stops that you may make while working your territory, depending upon the structure of your sales force and the types of products you sell.

Pharmacies. You will rarely *sell* to pharmacies, but pharmacists are essential resources for representatives in any territory. It's always useful to stop at selected retail pharmacies in your area to spend some time with the head pharmacists. These individuals are often very busy, however. To avoid annoying them, try to catch them at a time when traffic at the retail counter is slow.

When visiting a retail pharmacist:

- Ask about product "movement" off the shelves (regarding your company's products and the competition's).
- Inquire about trends…Does your product appear to be gaining or losing market share when compared with the competition?
- Try to find out which health plans (and physician group practices) are driving most of the business in your product's therapeutic category.
- Ask if patients are having any problems with administration, compliance, or side effects.
- Inquire about refill rates for chronic medications. (Low refill rates should be communicated to physicians who can, in turn, advise patients about the importance of refilling medications for chronic conditions.)
- Ask if the pharmacy is having any problems with product delivery, packaging, or general product quality.
- Ask for feedback about any special promotions associated with your products (for example, many companies offer special discounts for antibiotics if pharmacies agree to place orders in August or September, well in advance of cold and flu season).
- Ask if there is anything you or your company can do to make the pharmacist's job easier.

The stop-at-the-pharmacy strategy applies not just to retail pharmacies, but to hospital, clinic, and HMO pharmacies, too. In fact, at some hospitals and HMOs you may be required to check in with the pharmacy before you can visit physicians.

If you are new to a hospital, *always* stop at the pharmacy first to introduce yourself, identify the products that you are promoting, ensure that the pharmacy has current sales literature, and obtain guidelines for sales representative access. Always keep hospital and HMO pharmacies well stocked with promotional and clinical literature relating to your products.

Other customers

Again, depending upon the products that you sell and the structure of your sales force, you may be required to call on:
- government and Veterans Administration hospitals
- long-term care (LTC) and subacute care facilities
- home healthcare agencies
- prisons and jails (no kidding)

If these customers are on your call list, it will be essential for you to identify the unique needs of the populations within and to follow appropriate protocols regarding sales representative access and the promotion of pharmaceuticals. The appropriate manager within your company will provide you with the necessary resources and training for selling to these submarkets.

I used to call on an Air Force base in Massachusetts. The only difference between calling on military doctors and civilian doctors was that I addressed military physicians by their rank (e.g., "Captain Barnes," "Major Phillips") instead of "Doctor So-and-So."

I also routinely called on several Veterans Administration (VA) hospitals. Geriatric healthcare is usually the big focus in these institutions, but working a VA hospital is much the same as working any hospital.

The VA formulary (its list of approved drugs) is centralized nationally, but some VAs uses regional overrides. Pharmaceutical representatives joke that you can tell you are in a VA hospital with your eyes closed because many of the older patients (especially those from the World War II generation) smoke cigarettes.

VA hospitals utilize an enormous volume of prescription drugs, so if your product is on formulary and you can successfully "pull it through," you will have very little trouble making your numbers.

Nonphysician practitioners: NPs and PAs

In many healthcare settings nurse practitioners (NPs) and physician assistants (PAs) perform a variety of primary care functions. These individuals:

- take patient histories
- perform routine diagnostic and therapeutic procedures and physical exams
- diagnose colds, flu, and bacterial infections
- educate patients about preventive care, behavior modification, and prescription drugs

Because the services of these professionals cost less than physician services, the roles of NPs and PAs have grown dramatically in recent years. Many MCOs use nonphysician practitioners to provide screening and basic care for patients.

What's important for sales representatives is that these professionals enjoy prescribing privileges in nearly every state. Many NPs and PAs have excellent backgrounds in clinical pharmacology and often know more about pharmaceutical products than physicians do.

Both NPs and PAs can be influential with physicians and can be key "recommenders" regarding physician prescribing decisions. Generally, NPs and PAs are easier to see than physicians, too. Because NPs and PAs represent a relatively new and influential market, sales representatives should make it a point to win brand loyalty among NPs and PAs.

I can recall one group practice in which the doctors absolutely refused to see pharmaceutical representatives. However, I made it a point to cultivate a strong relationship with the office PA.

After awhile, the PA began advocating for my products among the physicians. He would always make sure that my samples were stocked and he would distribute literature for me. He would also discuss drug choices with the doctors and favorably position my company's products.

The bottom line is that the PA helped increase my products' market share despite the fact that I never interacted with any of the physicians at the practice. Eventually, I treated this particular PA just as I did any physician, inviting him to all my educational programs and physician social events.

A word about office staff

Although receptionists, office managers, and office nurses cannot prescribe medications, they represent potential allies in your efforts to see physicians and to help ensure that you secure and maintain prescription business at the office.

Receptionists are the office "gatekeepers." Their personalities can range from angelic to Attila the Hun-like. Believe me, I have seen the whole spectrum. Courtesy, friendliness, promptness, respect for waiting patients—and an occasional company give away—will help you build strong relationships with receptionists. When a receptionist is on your side, access to physicians is a lot easier.

I recall one receptionist in my territory who had an especially nasty disposition and—how can I say this kindly—she was the kind of lady whose appearance signals that the end of the opera is close at hand, if you catch my drift. She (I'll call her Gladys) snarled at me every time I showed up. I put on my best Eddie Haskell routine—"My, you're certainly looking great today, Gladys"—and killed her with kindness.

Eventually, she softened. As I got to know her, I discovered that her children represented the deepest passion in her life. Thereafter, I always made a point to ask about them and show her pictures of mine. Most competitive representatives completely gave up on the office because they considered her to be impenetrable. Finally, she arranged to let me see my targeted physician one day after hours. Sometimes success in selling takes this kind of special effort.

Make friends with office managers, too. The business side of health-care is just as important to physicians as the clinical side, and physicians entrust business operations to an office manager. Because cost and reimbursement issues influence the utilization of certain pharmaceuticals, it is often important to know the office manager at each practice on your call schedule.

This is not so important if you sell products that carry average price tags and are routinely reimbursed by insurance organizations. It *is* important if your product is expensive and not routinely covered. Certain oncology and radiopharmaceutical* products typically fall into these categories.

In these situations, the office manager will be a routine contact for you. In many cases, your job will simply be to advise the office manager of your company's reimbursement hotline, which, if available, is accessible by a toll-free phone call.

Office (and hospital) nurses are important contacts, too. Many nurses advise patients about administration of medications and are often familiar with patient histories. Some nurses may also function as second-line gatekeepers.

*   *   *   *   *

As I said at the beginning of the chapter, physicians are your most important customers. And whether you are face to face with a physician in a hospital or office setting, there is really no difference in how you handle your sales call. The next chapter takes a look at some of the basic selling skills that will help enhance your customer interactions.

---

* Radiopharmaceuticals refer to radioactive agents (e.g., radioactive iodine or cobalt) used for diagnostic or therapeutic purposes.

Chapter 7

Basic Selling Skills

It's time now to look at some of the basic skills and behaviors you must possess in order to be successful in pharmaceutical sales.

In the context presented here, "basic" refers to the common-sense skills and behaviors that all sales professionals must be able to demonstrate, regardless of the industry or product. I'll discuss these basic behaviors with a pharmaceutical spin. In Chapters 8 and 9, I'll focus on selling activities that are unique to pharmaceutical sales.

General professional behavior

Here's a story I often told when I was a sales trainer…

Imagine that you are single and have been admiring another certain single person for quite some time. Let's call this person Chris (a nice gender-neutral name). Chris is very attractive, intelligent, warm, witty, and fun to be with—the whole package. You have often thought about being with Chris in a significant way.

Now imagine that you have just had the worst workday of your life and you come home exhausted and in a totally rotten mood. As soon as you step into the house, the phone rings and you decide to answer it.

How would you respond if:

- the call is from your mother, who lives in the same neighborhood and asks if you can pick up a few grocery items and deliver them to her apartment that very evening
- the call is from Chris, who suggests that the two of you get together for dinner that very evening

Chances are that you would respond differently.

You may whine to your mother, "Mom, I've had a bad day, I just can't do it tonight. Please call another sibling."

With Chris, however, your response would probably be dramatically different "Hi, Chris. Thanks so much for calling...I had a pretty good day. Thanks for asking...Yes, I would *love* to have dinner together tonight...What time do you have in mind?"

The point I always make when I tell this story is that you have control over your attitude, mood, and behavior even when you may not think so. And just as it is in everyday life, so it is in pharmaceutical sales.

Therefore, regardless of what happened yesterday or on the previous call, when you are ready to enter a physician's office to promote your products, *choose* to have a positive, upbeat attitude. Some representatives naturally possess this attitude all the time anyway, so they don't have to make the choice at all. But if you are like me and your mood can sometimes shift with the wind direction, *choose* the proper mood before you step into the doctor's office.

This means that, regardless of what has happened up until the moment you greet the receptionist, you must remember to practice the following behaviors:

- Smile—a nice smile almost always wins friends and opens doors to physician offices.
- Remember first names of staff and ask how people are doing. Be sincere and listen to what they have to say. If your memory is shaky, write down what you learn in your physician profile, such as names and ages of children; new children and grandchildren in

the family; favorite hobbies, sports, and vacation places; favorite restaurants (very important if take-out is available for office lunches); and so on.

- Be courteous and respectful of what is going on around you. Patients always come first.
- If you tell the receptionist you will only require a few minutes of the physician's time, stick to your promise.
- Maintain an "attitude of gratitude." Say thank you for every small favor.
- Don't complain or criticize—assume that the customer's staff is always right (unless, for example, you are absolutely *certain* that the doctor is willing to see you when it looks like the receptionist is running interference).
- Observe pharmaceutical rep etiquette. Do not enter the office proper if another representative is already there. Remain in the waiting area until he or she leaves.

I am not suggesting that you put on phony airs or a plastic appearance. Above all, you must be yourself, and presumably you would not have been hired if anyone on the interview team detected any serious personality flaws. The fact that you are in this position indicates that you have a wonderful personality, you are intelligent and articulate, and possess personal attributes that people like. Your own positive "uniqueness" is a great selling point, so let it show.

Creating relationships with your customers (and their staff) in pharmaceutical sales is like building relationships with customers in any other line of selling. People buy the product, but and they *also* buy the salesperson.

How many times have you gone to a retail store, fully intending to buy a certain product but not doing so because the salesperson was unfriendly, unavailable, or unhelpful?

On the other hand, how many times have you entered a store with the idea of "just looking" but ended up buying an item that really cost more than what you planned to pay simply because the salesperson smiled, identified your needs, matched you up with a product, and went out of his or her way to confirm that this was exactly what you wanted in the first place?

Both scenarios happen every day in the sales world. Try to make certain that the *latter* scenario plays out in *your* day-to-day selling.

You're not sick!

Here's another point to keep in mind. Doctors see sick and unhappy people all day. They listen to complaints all the time.

*Very often, some physicians actually look forward to interacting with pharmaceutical representatives because you are **not** sick, unhappy, and complaining.*

A cheerful, friendly, representative allows for positive and engaging break in the physician's day.

Personal appearance

I'm not going to spend a lot of time on this. In the field you are expected to wear business dress, which means jacket-and-tie for men, and an appropriate suit, dress, or blouse-and-skirt combination for women. At most training and district meetings, business casual is acceptable, according to company policy. Visits to headquarters usually require business dress, but many companies have relaxed their dress codes in recent years.

Okay, I'm about to wander into a politically sensitive area, but what I am about to say needs to be said. It won't resonate among all of the women who read this—and I sincerely apologize if I offend you in any way. But, as I suggested above, this needs to be said–it may apply only to a few of you.

Female representatives should dress conservatively. I have observed new trainees in other modes of dress who have been pulled aside by male and female trainers alike to receive advice about these issues. It is an uncomfortable situation for everyone involved.

The simple solution is not to get in this situation to begin with. I understand there are cultural, generational, and gender differences but these really do not matter in the world of business. Your company is entitled to create and enforce dress codes. So, again, err on the side of caution. Be conservative.

Male representatives often get in trouble when they wear casual-looking sport coats or blazers in a business dress setting, or wear the wrong shoes (penny loafers) with suits.

Finally, I believe that every pharmaceutical sales representative should dress for success and be impeccably groomed, preferably on the *conservative* side. On occasions I have observed representatives who have dressed *too* fashionably. This is to say that wearing a $900 Armani suite or a Rolex watch may not sit too well with physicians and their office staff. My philosophy is that dress should say, "I'm a competent professional," not "I'm exceptionally well paid."

Here's a tip that you are unlikely to get anywhere else...

I noticed that after my first few days in the field, I came down with the cold or the flu or some other nasty affliction that knocked me out of com-mission—and commissions—for a few days. I have since discovered that many other rookie representatives had the same experience.

Here's why I think this happens: Dozens of sick people visit physician offices every day, spreading bacteria almost everywhere—doorknobs, coun-tertops, books and magazines, etc.

Prevailing medical opinion suggests that many bacterial infections are spread from hand-to-surface-to-hand-to-mouth, or some variation thereof—but hands are always in the mix. Consequently, so medical wisdom says, you can help prevent infections if you wash your hands regularly.

So reduce your risk. Imagine that you are Lady Macbeth. Wash your hands several times during the day.

You heard it here first.

Basic communication skills

All successful representatives possess above average communication skills, although not necessarily from the moment they are hired. Most new-hire training programs devote at least a day to communication basics, which include listening, questioning, reflecting, dealing with objections, and so on.

Here are some of my personal suggestions in these issues:

Avoid the "Robo-Rep" syndrome. Doctors hate "Robo-Reps." These are reps who deliver canned sales presentations exactly as if they were reading from a script. Okay, in your training programs when you are first learning how to do all this, you very well may be reciting from a script. That's acceptable in training.

In the real world, in front of customers, you need to get beyond this "presentation mode" and focus on "conversational level." Much has been made in contemporary sales training programs about the need to become a "consultative" representative. This means, that, instead of simply "pushing" products on physicians, you take the time to identify their real needs, then present solutions that match their needs.

To take it a step further, this means that you cannot simply enter a physician's office and launch into a carefully rehearsed script. Take the time to find out what the physician's concerns are regarding patients who are candidates for your product. In order to do this successfully, you must *ask good questions* and *be a good listener.*

Employ good questioning skills. You really can't sell anything to any-body—whether it's a pharmaceutical product or a household appliance—without first identifying the customer's needs. And the only way to identify needs is by *asking* about them, then *listening* to what the customer says in response. (I'll cover listening in a moment.)

For example, if a retail customer is in a department store checking out refrigerators, a savvy salesperson will not simply launch into a presentation about the ice-maker, the water dispenser, and the energy-saving thermostat. The customer might not care about any of these features. Instead, the salesperson might ask: "How much space do you have in your kitchen?", "What color do you prefer?", "What price range are you interested in?", and so on. Questions like these help the salesperson deliver a presentation that matches a customer's precise requirements for a refrigerator.

It's the same way with pharmaceuticals. A good sales representative will ask specific questions that direct the conversation toward the physician's prescribing needs regarding your product. These needs could relate to almost anything, for example, a need for:

- an easy dosing schedule
- a product with fewer side effects
- a medication that is safe to take with other medications
- a drug that can be safely taken by patients with high blood pressure
...and so on.

The point is, without getting answers to these questions, you might just as well deliver your presentation to a wall.

Virtually every selling skills program in the pharmaceutical industry includes questioning (or "probing") techniques, and each company seems to have its own spin on methods and terminology.

I won't get into specific methods here. My point is, during every sales call, always ask a few questions to identify customer needs. The responses provide you with prompts that will help you complete a successful call.

Be a good listener. This may very well be the most important skill a representative can employ. Yet it is surprising how many representatives (and how many of us in general) are poor listeners. Time and time again in selling skills workshops, trainers stage introductory listening exercises designed to test listening skills, and invariably, a fairly high percentage of participants fail.

You don't have to take sales training programs to practice good listening skills. You can work on this skill in everyday life when interacting with family, friends, store clerks, and fellow employees.

One good way to sharpen listening skills is to practice the related skill of paraphrasing. For example, in a sales situation, you might reflect on what a doctor has just said by saying something like, "Doctor, if I understand you correctly, a fairly high percentage of patients who are taking Drug X are complaining about drowsiness. Is that correct?"

Reflecting helps you confirm that you understand what the customer said and provides you with a starting point to explain an advantage of your product.

Other communication skills include such basics as maintaining eye contact, using your sales aid as a focal point for discussion, pausing for effect after making a key benefit statement, and acknowledging a physician's concerns and objections regarding your product.

Building rapport

Sometimes, physicians on your call list will become personal friends. This does not happen very often, nor should it even be a goal with every physician. Your professional goal is to encourage every physician you call on to prescribe your company's products.

My point is, when you become friends with a physician, you have succeeded at developing a high level of rapport. These are physicians with whom you can talk comfortably about almost any subject, and where the informal banter flows easily.

Rapport occurs at many levels. You can, over time, establish rapport even with gruff, impatient, hard-to-see physicians. With these physicians, you'll generally maintain a strictly professional relationship, which is fine.

Over time, you will develop a sort of "sixth sense" regarding the appropriate level of rapport you develop with each individual physician.

As suggested earlier, rapport is important with office staff and nurses, too. These individuals often wield considerable influence over access to physicians, so develop relationships with these individuals, too.

Create a goal for *every* call

One way in which some representatives fall down on the job is that they fail to set a goal for *every* sales call. It's one thing to have weekly, monthly, quarterly, and annual goals. But some representatives just make calls on physicians with no objective other than to simply get some face time with the doctor. That is not enough.

Before you enter the office on a call, it's important to have a very specific goal in mind. Examples might include:

- Introduce a new product.
- Ask the physician to read a clinical paper.
- Determine the physician's results with your sampling program.
- Restock the sample closet.
- Secure a commitment to prescribe your product.
- Invite the physician to be a guest speaker.
- Gain a commitment for the physician to attend a medical education event sponsored by your company.
- Ask the physician to recommend your product to other physicians.

These goals apply to *all* calls, even "30-second" encounters with physicians in corridors and elevators. (You'll learn more about these calls in the next chapter.)

Goals can be "big" or "small." It doesn't matter, as long as you continue to advance the physician toward becoming a "champion" for your product. Sometimes this can occur in a few months. In other cases, it will take years. But if you create goals along the way, it will be easier for you to track your own progress from month-to-month.

The skills I have just outlined represent the plain-vanilla basics. Every company puts its own spin on how to train you to develop these skills. Regardless of how you learn and practice them, you will need to execute them on every sales call.

Speaking of sales calls, let's see what they are all about...

Chapter 8

The Sales Call

You're probably wondering, what does a pharmaceutical sales representative actually *do* when he or she enters a physician's office and promotes a prescription drug. That's a very good question. I had no idea what a typical sales call was like until I began my training. And even after training, I had no real idea what a typical call was like. That's because when I went out into the field I discovered that there is *no such thing* as a typical sales call in this business.

The fact is, every sales call is different, with its own unique goal (see previous chapter), pace, ebb and flow, and result. Still, you need to have some idea regarding the structure of a sales call, so this chapter provides you with an overview.

Keep in mind that each company teaches the structure of a call in a different manner, but essentially, every call requires:

- Pre-call planning
- An opener
- A feature/benefit presentation
- Opportunities for questions and objections
- A close

• Post-call analysis

Let's see how this plays out in a standard office call.

Pre-call planning

Every call requires planning. Without it, you're simply running on a treadmill. Here are some questions that work well in the pre-call planning process:

• Is this a first-time visit to the physician?
• What did we talk about on my last visit?
• Did I set expectations on my last call? If so, how can I fulfill them today?
• Do I need to provide responses to unanswered questions or objections that came up during the last call?
• What does my company data show about this physician's prescribing habits?
• With which managed care plans is this physician affiliated?
• What are the physician's outside interests, activities, hobbies, etc.? (in case you need ideas for an opener).
• What is sales representative protocol for this practice?
• What is my goal for this call?

Go over all of these issues while driving to the next call. Focus on the goal of the call, and rehearse the call in your mind (even though the call will never proceed precisely as rehearsed).

Before you see the doctor…

Doctors are busy and cannot always see you on a moment's notice. If you must wait, here are a couple of suggestions on how to maximize your time:

Ask a nurse or office manager appropriate questions about the practice and your product.

Let your eyes roam—you'll collect lots of hints about a doctor's education, hobbies, travel interests, family life, etc., just by looking at photos, artwork, and so on.

On this last point, a popular activity originally conducted by training guru Bob Pike is a great way to sharpen your observation skills. In the activity, everyone is instructed to draw the front and back sides of a US penny from memory, without help.

At the same time trainees are asked to estimate how many pennies they have actually handled over their lifetimes. Guesses ran into the hundreds of thousands.

The portraits of Honest Abe are always hilarious and not very accurate. Few renderings of the pennies are anywhere close to being accurate.

Then, participants are asked to share each other's portraits and fill in missing items that the other representatives may have missed.

One lesson related to the exercise is this: Very often there is a wealth of information directly in front of you (or in your pocket) that you miss simply because you've never taken the time to look. In the case of pharmaceutical selling, look around the office and learn. Then **apply** *your knowledge during the sales call.*

Another lesson is that the exercise demonstrates the value of teamwork. You may often co-promote a product with a colleague who visits the same customer. This individual may know things that you do not. If you share information about the customer, each of you has the opportunity to obtain some valuable information that can help you win the business.

Opening the call

Every call needs an opener, something to break the ice and establish rapport between the sales representative and the physician.

The first time you meet a physician, don't launch into a presentation unless he or she asks something like, "What have you got for me today?"

Common sense says that you should introduce yourself, identify your company, name the product you are about to promote, and explain that you are present to serve the *doctor's* needs by providing information, about your company's products, and services.

I remember my first few weeks in the field. I was excited to tell doctors everything I knew about my product. I recall my first real presentation. It was at the end of my first day (no one would see me all that day, despite numerous stops). It was about 6 p.m. and I waited a long time to see the doctor because the receptionist assured me that he would give me some time.

Finally, my big moment…I was nervous but very determined. We shook hands and I took out my sales aid and launched into the presentation, head down, page by page, by page. Fifteen minutes later with a kindly smile on his face, the doctor said, "You're new at this, huh?" I mumbled something like, "Yeah. How can you tell?"

All he *really* wanted to know on that particular call was: Who was I? Did I replace another representative? What product was I promoting? Did I have any *new* information for him?

He most definitely did not want the "Robo-Rep" that I presented myself to be. He wanted a conversation, not a commercial presentation.

Fortunately, he was a nice guy and I learned a lot on that call. At that time of day, he could have booted me out of the office and gone home.

So, then, to open a call you must first *break the ice*. Any topic will do (weather, current events, etc.), but the more personal the better (hobbies, the physician's family, local medical events, etc.).

You will have planned the call, so you know what you want to focus on and what objectives you would like to achieve. Therefore, you must follow your opener with something that is going to point you in that general direction.

The next step in your opener is to focus on a particular need of the physician, which will allow you make the transition into your actual presentation.

For example, you might say something like, "Doctor, the last time we spoke you mentioned that you see a lot of elderly patients who notice side effects quite easily and that these patients are tough to keep on medications over the long term. The great news is that a recent 12-month study demonstrated that Drug X, when evaluated in an elderly patient population, showed superior efficacy and also high tolerability. This will allow you to treat your patients over the long run."

This approach provides the doctor with a good reason to listen to you. It gains the doctor's attention because it is tailored to his/her needs and concerns. Always prepare a tailored opening during precall planning.

Features and benefits

You'll hear these terms so often during training that you'll tire of them rapidly, but it is essential that you understand how features and benefits fit into professional sales.

When I conducted training programs, I used to ask participants to imagine themselves as real estate salespeople. Suppose you were trying to sell a typical three-bedroom cape-style home with a big yard and a finished basement. These are features—descriptors of the product.

I would then divide the class into two groups and ask each group to come up with benefit statements to match each household feature. I instructed Group 1 to assume that they would show the house to a young family, and told Group 2 that the prospects were an elderly retired couple.

The results were amazing. You would never know that both groups were showing the same house!

Take a look at the responses:

Feature—"Big Yard"

- Group 1 (Family)–Children will have room to play sports such as soccer or wiffle-ball.

- Group 2 (Couple)–Lots of room to install the shuffle
board game that the couple loved on cruises.
Feature—"Finished Basement"
- Group 1 (Family)–Parents will have a place for kids
and toys, producing less noise and clutter in the main
living area.
- Group 2 (Couple)–Extra storage for antiques the couple has been collecting over the years.

You get the picture. The same features can translate into several different benefits depending upon the *audience* and its unique *needs*.

Let's shift to pharmaceuticals. Pharmaceuticals deliver benefits to several audiences: patients, providers, and the community, and each of these audiences can be subdivided into several niche audiences.

- Patients: Young patients. Male patients. Female patients. Young female patients. Elderly patients. Patients who smoke. You name it. Your presentation may thus need to focus on benefits for specific groups, and the benefits may not be identical among groups.
- *Providers*: Providers are typically physicians, but you can also create specific benefit messages for healthcare providers such as pharmacists, nurses, office staff, residents, etc.
- *Community:* This can be the hospital or managed care community or even the healthcare community in general. You can even think big and include society in general.

My point is, you can promote the same product to all three broad audiences and to each niche audience, and your benefit messages may be different for each audience. Features and benefits for pharmaceutical products generally focus on four areas:

- *Efficacy*–Does the product work, and, if so, how well?
- *Safety*–Can patients take the drug with little or no concern about possible side effects?
- *Convenience*–Is the product easy to administer? Can a patient take it once a day instead of three or four times?

- *Cost*–Is it less expensive than similar medications? If it costs more, do I get better value?

Sales calls should address features and benefits in all of these areas, but avoid overload. I worked with a training colleague who always said, "When you go fishing you don't need to put the whole worm on the hook to catch a fish, just a small piece of the worm." Similarly, in pharmaceutical sales, you don't need to go through 20 minutes of features and benefits for a physician. A few carefully selected items *based on the physician's needs* should work perfectly.

A typical drug feature is generally accompanied by one or two clearly identifiable benefits. For example, "Doctor, Drug X has no drug interactions (FEATURE). This means that your elderly patients will be able to take it with any other medication without worry (BENEFIT 1), and you will happy because the efficacy of all the medications will not be compromised (BENEFIT 2)."

Sounds easy enough, doesn't it. But your feature-and-benefit presentation simply sets you up for dealing with…

Questions and objections

It's hard enough to learn all the scientific information, selling skills, features and benefits, and how to use sales aids. But after practice, you become quite capable. Then the problem is, "Oh my gosh, the doctor asked me a question," or "Uh-oh, he's objecting to something I just said."

Typically, newly hired representatives come up with a deer-in-the-headlights look and stare at the doctor thinking, "But that's not in the script." Actually, questions and objections *are* in the script, and you will be well trained on how to deal with them. Market research with physician "focus groups" reveals well in advance of a product's launch exactly what types of questions physicians will ask about the product and how they might object to what you say. Role play after role play in training sessions will help prepare you for this part of the call.

When you think about it, whenever a physician expresses a question, concern, or outright objection, it simply presents you with another opportunity to promote the advantages of your product. It's an opportunity to *sell* because your customer's questions are a sign that he or she is *engaged* in the discussion and has invited you into a dialogue!

Your responsibility is to *acknowledge* the physician ("Doctor, that's a good point you raise"), and then to provide the information that addresses the issue.

What's an objection? It's a physician concern that may represent a roadblock to prescriptions. It can be as simple as a question such as "How much does it cost?", or it can be expressed as outright worry such as, "Frankly, I'm worried about the side effects of this product."

You need to take care to probe for the rationale behind an objection. Consider the following interaction in the middle of a sales call:

Doctor: How much does your drug cost?

Representative: It's only costs about a dollar a day, doctor.

Doctor: Thanks. What else do you have for me today?

The likely result? You continue the call and the physician does not prescribe your product.

Why did the doctor *not* prescribe the product? After all you were honest and provided the answer that he/she was looking for, didn't you? Not really.

Perhaps you did not realize that the doctor was comparing your product's price to the price of another product that he or she routinely prescribes. It's easy to avoid problems by responding with an open-ended question.

In this example, you might say something like, "Doctor, that's a very good question. What therapies are you comparing to?"

The doctor's response to a question like this will usually provide you with all sorts of useful information suggesting what is important to the doctor, who might say to you, "Well, I actually prescribe diuretics most of the time and they are pretty inexpensive for my patients."

Now you know what you are really dealing with. The doctor is concerned about cost for "the patients" and that the doctor prescribes a lot of diuretic medications. You can then continue by comparing your product with diuretics, hopefully with a reliable clinical study that analyzes the products head-to-head.

Here, then, are the rules of thumb for handling objections:

- Acknowledge the physician's concern.
- Probe to determine the cause of the concern.
- Respond with at least one feature and benefit.
- Close the loop by confirming that you have addressed the physician's concern.

When you address objections in this manner, you'll find that objection-handling is just another fun and fascinating part of selling.

Closing the call

To close a call, first return to your goal. Was it to gain the physician's commitment to prescribe? To read a clinical paper? To participate in an event?

Your close should be a request to secure a physician's commitment that is aligned with the goal of the call.

The Robo-Rep's close is always the same: "So doctor, will you put all you patients on Drug X and prescribe it for everyone with [whatever the disease or condition is] in the future?"

But you are not Robo-Rep. My point is that you have to close appropriately. If you have done a good job with well-targeted features and benefits, and if the doctor has never tried the drug before, ask the doctor to *try* it. If the doctor has already prescribed it, ask if he or she will try it in other patient types.

Another point to remember about closing is to state the product's name and proper dose. The dose is a product's "last name," so to speak. You do not want the doctor to prescribe too much or too little of your product for a particular patient type. If that happens, the doctor may form an opinion that the drug does not work (if the dose is too low) or that the side effects are too risky (if the dose is too high).

Remember, when closing, you are trying to help the physician make a decision. You want the doctor to be confident in prescribing the product for all the right reasons—the *doctor's* reasons, not yours.

In other words, eliminate the attitude that you close for *your* benefit. Instead, adopt the approach that you close for the *physician's* benefit and for their *patients'* benefit. You close for the organizations that they work for and with. You are in the field to meet *their* needs, not yours.

Post-call analysis

When you get back to your car after a call, *write down* key information (or enter it in your laptop computer) that summarizes what you achieved—or did not achieve—during the call.

This may include:
- status of samples in the sample closet and number of samples left today
- the title of a clinical journal you may have left behind
- the physician's current attitude about your product, and whether or not he or she agreed to prescribe it
- action items (such as a date to schedule the next call, or following up on a commitment to provide certain information)

Your post-call analysis then becomes the first item to check when performing pre-call planning for the next call.

Be brief. Be bright. Be gone.

I want to wrap up the sales call section by focusing on the principle that guided me throughout my sales career: Be brief. Be bright. Be gone.

Be brief. Your presentations should be well thought out in advance. Features and benefits should be targeted to physicians needs, concerns, and patient types. Focus *only* on a physician's stated needs.

You may be having a great conversation with the doctor about last night's ball game, or even about the latest in invasive cardiovascular surgery techniques, but if you take too long either the doctor or the nurse is going to give you hints that you should be moving on. Don't develop a reputation of taking up too much of a physician's time. You will not be welcome for future visits. If the doctor says you only have five minutes, then stick to the five-minute limit.

Be bright. Sales representative credibility is critical in this business. You need to demonstrate that you are knowledgeable about clinical issues, patient needs, managed care, office protocol, you name it. You *must* have the ability to hold fairly high-level conversations with your customers. Believe me, I have spoken to plenty of physicians who have told me about representatives who just didn't know their stuff. These representatives rarely earn a physician's business.

Be gone: Doctors and their staffs are busy. Managed care rules often dictate that they must see as many patients as they can during the day and that they observe efficient time-management practices. You may be a wonderful, warm, intelligent, and witty person, but you also represent precious *time* to some physicians. Some physicians will not see you for this reason alone. Don't take it personally. Be grateful for those physicians who do see you, and *respect their time.*

If you follow the 3 Be's on every call, you should discover that, over time, your "Be gone" time will be extended with certain physicians, and you will have more opportunities to promote your products.

The "30-second sales call"

So far, we've talked about the office call, which might last five minutes or so. And we've advised you to be brief, be bright, and be gone.

What do you do when you have a mere *30 seconds* to capture a physician's attention? Do you just say hello and move on?

Never. Every day representatives "connect" with their physician customers in 30 seconds or less. Mastering the 30-second call (or, in some circles, the "abridged call") is just another skill that you will learn in training. With practice and experience, you will become an expert at these quick calls.

The fact of the matter is that no matter how well known you are and no matter how friendly or well liked by physicians, there will be many times when customers simply do not have time to speak with you.

Don't take it personally. Doctors and nurses do have other responsibilities…such as treating patients! And although they may not have time to speak to you, chances are, you *do* have time to speak to them. So *take advantage of the opportunity!*

Here's a typical scenario: A sales representative meets Dr. Brown in a hospital corridor…

> *Representative:* "Good morning Dr. Brown. I've been looking forward to my visit with you today"
> *Dr. Brown:* "Sorry, Laura, I don't have time to talk today. I just got called to the ER."

Or, another representative encounters Dr. Green checking a patient's record at the receptionist's counter…

> *Representative:* "Hello, Dr. Green. I'm here for my 2:30 appointment."
> *Dr. Green:* "Oh, I'm sorry, Rick. I have a staff meeting at the hospital in 15 minutes and I've scheduled an extra patient before I leave. It will have to wait for another day."

So what do you do?

Remember: Time equals money. The more time you can spend talking about your product with a customer, the more likely it is that he or she will prescribe it. Clearly, however, you can see in above situations that attempting to consume your customer's time in any significant way would not be in anyone's best interest. You must consider the Golden Rule in these situations, or you may never get any time with the customer in the future.

The solution, of course, is the abridged presentation. Mention your product's name and hand the physician a copy of your sales aid. Remind the physician of an important feature, such as a new dose or a new formulation…and be gone.

Here's another tactic: Let's say that a receptionist tells you firmly that Dr. Black cannot see you today. In this situation, you might ask to check to see if the sample cabinet needs restocking with your product. Tell the receptionist that you will need to obtain a signature from the doctor but you will not take more than a minute or so of Dr. Black's time.

Then, once you make your promise, keep it! The physician *and* the receptionist will remember your actions, and they will learn to trust you.

Creativity leads to a 30-second call

*I once called on a cardiology practice that moved its office to a new location. On my first visit the receptionist told me that I could absolutely not see the doctor. (I could see why—he **did** have a packed waiting room.)*

After engaging in small talk about the move and the new office, I learned that the sample closet was not set up yet and they were not looking forward to doing it. Intuitively, I volunteered for the job on the spot. It only took about an hour to unpack all the boxes and arrange the products on the shelves. My efforts even led to an abridged presentation with one of the cardiologists.

When I finished the job, the staff was so happy about the skillful organization of the closet that they said I would be the only representative allowed to access the closet. It was, after all, my creation.

The bottom line is: Don't be afraid to roll up your sleeves to help out the office staff. It's a great way to enhance relations with the staff, and you might even secure some unanticipated time with a doctor.

Tips for 30-second calls

Here are some suggestions on how to successfully complete a 30-second call:

- Always be prepared with sales literature or a clinical reprint to present to the physician.
- Open with a statement about the product's unique feature, or about a *new* feature (a newly approved dose), or about an issue that addresses a physician's need (which you may know from a prior call).
- Choose one page or "spread" of your literature to support the point you make in step 2.
- Emphasize benefits—for the physician (e.g., no dose adjustments required), for patients (e.g., fast-acting), or both.
- Close for a commitment, as described earlier in this chapter.

If you sense that you can buy more time and the situation allows it, simply ask an open ended question or two; questions that demands something other than a "yes" or "no" answer. By asking the customer to express his or her feelings about a clinical topic, or to analyze, compare, or contrast treatment protocols, you suddenly find yourself in a conversation. With this conversation comes information which you can use to provide product solutions.

The "Match" Game

When teaching abridged presentations trainers sometimes pass out long wooden matches. They instruct representatives to pair up, one playing the role of representative; the other, the physician. When the trainer says "Go," the representative playing the doctor lights the match. The goal for the presenting representative is to open, present a few well-chosen benefits, and close before the customer gets "burned." Burn the customer and you burn your chances for a return visit.

I often required representatives to make many abridged presentations during their training programs. At any time the trainers were fair-game "doctors"—in hallways, parking lots, and even the dining rooms!

How to see "no-see" physicians

"No-see" physicians are physicians who, ostensibly, refuse to see sales representatives. In reality, there are several techniques savvy representatives employ in order to secure face time with these tough-to-see physicians.

One of my district managers told me, "There is a marked difference between a comfortable representative and wealthy representative." What he meant is that successful representatives often need to expand their comfort zones. They need to be more assertive and creative, especially when it comes to customers that, for one reason or another, don't want to see pharmaceutical representatives.

Here is a list of ideas that can help promote interactions with no-see physicians.

- *See the doctor in the hospital instead of in the office.* In the hospital, although he or she needs to visit patients and attend conferences, a doctor generally has fewer time restraints than when in the office. Also, you avoid receptionists who try to protect the doctors' schedules. Plus, if a no-see physician observes you inter-acting with peers, he or she may thereafter deem it "OK" to speak with you.

- *"Romance" the gatekeeper:* Be exceptionally nice and distribute lots of your nicer premium items to receptionists. If over the course of time you can make their life easier they may become strong allies. Perform well in this area and you may be the only representative allowed to see the physician.

- *Invite the doctor to a speaker program:* A little ego massage never hurts, so send a note asking a no-see physician to participate in one of your company's speaker programs. Or ask him or her to attend a program at which one of his esteemed colleagues is pre-senting. You never know what might draw the physician out of the office. It could be a hot clinical topic, a well-known speaker, or even the new restaurant in town. Whatever it is, once these doctors are out of the office and in a social setting, they often open up to conversation. This is your opportunity to let them know that you are a resource.

- *Provide "new" information:* Some no-see physicians think repre-sentatives deliver the "same-old-same-old" information. However, if you are promoting a breakthrough product, or a product with a new indication, or have a landmark clinical study, then you may be awarded an audience with the physician.

- *At Hospital Displays:* To set up your company's display you often have to arrange for a time and a place with a hospital or clinic. Depending on the date and time, yours may be the only display in the doctor's lounge. On the other hand, you may be one of several displays outside a hospital conference auditorium.

- *Send a letter:* You are usually not allowed to communicate in writ-ing about your company or its products unless you use officially sanctioned company literature, including direct mail letters. If your company provides these letters, take advantage of them and mail them to your customers. These letters often state that you will be more than happy to meet to discuss the information or provide product samples. When a physician responds, you have a ticket to see the doctor.

- *Send a birthday card:* Asking good questions to gatekeepers often results in information such as a physician's birthday. Small courtesies such as a birthday card help ensure that a physician remembers you the next time he or she sees your business card.
- *Page the doctor at the hospital:* Yes, this takes assertiveness but more often than not it pays off. The key to your success is that when the doctor answers your page is to be friendly and straightforward. "Doctor, I'm David Currier from SuperPharm and I would like to meet over a cup of coffee when you are free today to learn more about your clinical practice. I also have some information that may have a beneficial effect on many of your patients." Very often, the response will be, "Sure, meet me in the cafeteria in half an hour." Always thank the physician for responding to your page and meeting with you.
- *Take the customer golfing:*....if, of course, golf is part of your company's culture and the physician is a golfer. This is a great opportunity to socialize with a physician who might otherwise not spend time with you.
- *Volunteer with local patient advocacy groups:* Many physicians are regularly involved with groups such as the Arthritis Foundation or the Diabetes Foundation for fundraising and educational purposes. Become involved with a group that deals with patients your product treats or with a group you find personally rewarding.

Above all, think creatively. A colleague of mine once mailed four playing cards to a no-see doc. Later, he showed up at the physician's office with a fifth card which, together with the original four, created a royal straight flush. He handed the fifth card and his business card (with a small note written on it) to the receptionist, who then gave to the doctor.

The "card trick" worked. The physician called the representative and invited him to the office. Why did it work? Because the representative learned from another physician that this particular doctor had a passion for poker, an interest shared by the representative. From that point on, the representative became part of the doctor's regular poker group, played in monthly games and, oh, yes…got to see the doctor whenever he wanted to.

*   *   *   *   *

In this chapter, I have described the "typical" sales call, told you how to complete a 30-second call, and provided tips on how to get to know "no-see" docs. Throughout the chapter, I mentioned sales literature, clinical studies, samples, and so on. All of these items are, at one time or another, essential for supporting the call. The next chapter takes a closer look at how to use these items.

Chapter 9

Supporting the Sales Call

Very few, if any, sales calls stand on their own without supportive literature and clinical data. I mentioned in Chapter 4 that it would be necessary for you to organize and store a wide variety of documents. Now it's
time to take these documents out of storage and examine how to use
them to support your selling messages.

We'll take a look at three types of documents that support your efforts
on most calls: the sales aid, the package insert, and the clinical paper.
We'll also look at another key sales support activity: product sampling.

The sales aid

The sales aid (sometimes called a "detail aid" or "visual aid") is the
principal promotional document you will use to support your selling
messages. Most sales aids are glossy, full-color documents, produced by
an advertising agency (under the direction of the marketing department), usually measuring 8½″ x 11″.

Page count varies. Four pages is the minimum (an 11″ x 17″ sheet of
heavy-duty paper stock folded in half). Eight or 12 pages are probably
standard lengths for these documents. Sometimes, sales aids feature a

pocket inside the back cover where you can insert a clinical paper, a package insert, and a business card.

Sales aids serve a couple of purposes. First, they provide you with a visual focus for your sales presentation. Although you should never *read* from a sales aid, your ability to point to key headlines or graphics with a pen reinforces your verbal cues and provides a focal point for the customer.

Second, several sales aids are perfect "leave-behind" pieces. They provide the physician with a permanent reference/reminder about the product. They also provide you with a useful reference point when opening your next sales call, ("Doctor, the last time I was here, I provided you with the Product X product brochure...")

Sales aids are usually organized in the following manner:

Cover page. A cover page often features an appropriate photograph, along with a headline that effectively positions the product (e.g., "First combination therapy for blood pressure with once-daily dosing").

Features and benefits. The next several pages focus on key features and benefits, usually starting with efficacy, followed by safety, then convenience.

Efficacy features usually focus on a product's mechanism of action, fast-acting (or long-lasting) capability, proven results in trials, or head-to-head performance with another leading brand. Efficacy claims are usually supported with charts and graphs extracted from clinical trial data.

Safety features generally come next, although, if a favorable side-effect profile is the product's top selling feature, safety may come first. On the safety pages, you will find data regarding a product's adverse events profile.

For example, current medications in a certain therapeutic category may be noted for a particularly common adverse event (or side effect), say, nausea. If trials with your product show a low incidence of nausea, then a headline in the safety section of the sales aid may emphasize that fact.

A sales aid also includes a table listing side effects reported among 2% or more of subjects in clinical trials. The table compares the frequency of side effects reported by patients taking the advertised medication against the percentages reported among patients taking a placebo (a "dummy" pill or capsule containing no active ingredient). Typical side effects for commonly prescribed drugs include nausea, dizziness, diarrhea, dry mouth, and headache.

Convenience features and benefits relate to dosing and administration. The sales aid will usually promote such benefits as "once-a-day dosing" or "two convenient doses" or "no titration required." (Titration refers to the process whereby a physician starts a patient on a low dose of a medication to assess efficacy and possible side effects, then switches to a higher dose to ensure greater efficacy.)

Summary page. A sales aid usually concludes with a summary page that highlights key information presented in the preceding pages. Reference to the summary page is a good way to wrap up your presentation before soliciting questions from a physician.

Sales aids may address cost benefits of your product from time to time, perhaps including a general statement that the product is "cost-effective therapy." Companies do not want representatives focusing on price with physicians, so price is not referenced in the sales aid, and you will not normally discuss price during sales calls. Your product's local price is subject to change on short notice, as is the price of competitive products. The proper forum for price discussions is the negotiation between national account managers and their customers. Your job is to focus on how your product represents value—in terms of reduced hospital stays or reduced need for other medications.

Back-up sales aids. Very often, the principal sales aid is "backed up" by a smaller piece for use as reminders on follow-up visits. The smaller pieces usually focus on the unique characteristics of a product and summarize efficacy, safety, and dosing information.

The back-up pieces may be produced as "slim jims" (pocket-sized 8½" x 3½" brochures) or a single, two-sided 8½" x 11" sheet printed on both sides.

Use binders for multi-product presentations

Most representatives promote several products and carry a sales-aid binder that organizes selling sheets by product in order of the product's importance. This is usually a thin (½- inch) three-ring binder with top-loading glycene sheets into which the product sheets are inserted.

This arrangement allows the representative to tell a story that connects all the products. This is accomplished through effective "bridging" from product to product. During quarterly sales meetings, your district managers will advise you on how to carefully craft these multi-product stories.

Be careful on multi-product calls. Your objective is to clinically convince the physician that his or her decision to prescribe your product is a rational one. Be sure that when promoting multiple products that you do not dilute the message of any one product in your portfolio. Selling multiple products works best when each product is positioned within a larger, related context.

The package insert

You learned in Chapter 4 that a package insert (PI) is a small, multi-fold informational brochure that includes all relevant prescribing information (and a lot more) about every product. The federal Food and Drug Administration (FDA) requires this type of "product labeling" for all prescription drug products.

You'll recall that a PI features highly detailed clinical information about a product including chemical composition, mechanism of action (how the active ingredient works), clinical pharmacology, pharmacokinetics, indications, contraindications, clinical study summaries, adverse event profiles, warnings and precautions, drug interactions, dosing and administration, and packaging.

Key information from the package insert is always presented in the sales aid, but physicians may have detailed questions about the product and you may need to reference the PI during a sales call.

Some marketing campaigns require representatives to leave the PI on every sales call. Some companies reproduce PI data directly in the sales aid. Others direct sales representatives to insert the PI in the back pocket of the sales aid.

A few words about the PI

The package insert is designed as a reference tool for physicians. It is not a sales aid or a promotional piece. With that in mind, if you must refer to the PI during a sales call, don't ever read from it. You should be familiar enough with it so that you can paraphrase it instead.

If you are using the PI as a visual aid, point to the headlines. Remember, too, that your sales aid may cover the same information as the PI in a more visually appealing format. So use the sales aid when possible.

Never use a yellow marker to highlight key passages in the PI (or any other literature, including clinical reprints). It is very tempting to do this, especially if the PI presents unique data highly advantageous to your product. Unfortunately, FDA regulations prohibit this type of product marketing.

*Remember: Key data from the PI is always highlighted in the **sales aid**.*

Clinical studies

Before a pharmaceutical product can be marketed in the United States, it must undergo a rigorous series of tests or "clinical trials"— from initial testing on laboratory animals to extensive "Phase IV" clinical trials involving hundreds or thousands of human subjects.

Even after a product is successfully launched, pharmaceutical manufacturers may invest hundreds of millions of dollars in comparative trials. In these trials, one drug is tested head-to-head against a competitive product to determine which one, if either, is faster- (or longer-) acting, has fewer side effects, has a higher cure rate, and so on.

Most of these studies are published in medical journals, and reprints of these studies represent highly effective and credible sales tools because they usually provide objective information about your products.

Terminology varies among pharmaceutical companies. Some companies simply refer to these studies as "reprints." Other terms include "clinical reprints," "journal articles," and "clinical papers." Regardless of what you call them, every sales representative's car (and home storage area) is well stocked with them, and their purpose is to provide clinically sound, statistically reliable, objective data about a product's performance among real patients.

What one physician says about clinical studies

"I think that the glossy brochures are nice to look at but they tend to be more marketing material. I think it's also important for representatives to show the studies that support the brochures. It's a matter of credibility. A study shows us that there is more than just the company that's behind the drug."

—Andrew Kriegel, MD
CardiologistBrockton,
Massachusetts

From "Reprint Ready," Total Learning Concepts, Inc, © 1999.

When I was in the field, I discovered that journal articles provide varying degrees of credibility, depending upon their source. After a few months of selling, I learned that I could mentally sort journal articles into three categories: "Highly Respected," "Respected," and "Throw Away."

In my world view (others are free to disagree), the best example of a "Highly Respected" journal is probably *The New England Journal of Medicine.* You often hear it quoted in the media regarding new revelations about diet or heart disease or cancer or other "hot" medical issues. "The Journal" is considered top-notch because its articles are subject to stringent peer review by highly respected "Ivory Tower" physicians. Several physician specialties have their own journals in my Highly Respected category. A good example is the *Journal of the American College of Cardiology,* or "JACC."

Generally speaking, I've found that physicians seem to pay closer attention to articles that originate in the "Highly Respected" category.

My "Respected" category features journals that have somewhat less stringent entry requirements. They are peer reviewed and the articles will capture the attention of physicians, but a little extra "sell" may be required to ensure that physicians read a reprint that supports your product. A respected journal in this category might be *The Journal of the American Medical Association (JAMA)* or *The Lancet.*

When you present a "Throw Away" article, a physician is likely to do just that with it. Studies that are analyzed in these articles are generally funded exclusively by a pharmaceutical manufacturer (which, by FDA law, must be so noted in the article), are not generally peer reviewed, and may have less rigorous study designs.

I have supported product sales with all three types of studies and, regardless of its source, a well-designed, credible, study will almost always capture a physician's attention.

Profile of a clinical study

Clinical studies almost always follow the same format, which makes them relatively easy to skim in order to obtain critical information. Skimming is okay when you first look at a study, but, if you are supporting a product with a study, *always* read the entire study and highlight key information *in your own personal copy* for you own personal reference. Never highlight a study for handing over to a physician—it is against FDA regulations to do so.

Wading through a lengthy study takes some time and effort. You'll encounter a lot of complicated medical statistics, but you must be an expert on your product and on all the studies that support its benefits. Whenever you see a study for the first time, set aside 45 minutes to an hour of quiet time—in your office, den, or on the deck—along with your favorite hot or cold beverage, and a yellow highlighter.

Here is what you will find:

Title/author. The title provides an overview of what the study is all about. Sometimes the titles themselves take a while to read.

An example of a study title is "Screening and Treatment for Cardiovascular Disease in Patients with Chronic Renal Disease."

Here's another example—one of my favorites…(take a deep breath)…: "A Preliminary Study of the Effects of Correction of Anemia With Recombinant Human Erythropoietin Therapy on Sleep, Sleep Disorders, and Daytime Sleepiness in Hemodialysis Patients." Fortunately, this study has its own acronym, the "SLEEPO" study, which makes it easier for sales representatives to refer to when discussing it with physicians.

The title is immediately followed by the authors' names. I say authors because most studies feature multiple authors, with the lead researcher's name coming first. If the study's name is too long to remember, it's common practice to refer to the study by the principal author's name. Hence, a study authored by Doctors Brown, Green, Black, Gray, and Redd, would normally be referred to as the "Brown Study."

Authors' names can be important to a targeted physician, especially if the principal author resides high up in the Ivory Tower and is well-known within his or her specialty.

Abstract. The abstract comes next and provides an "executive summary" of the material featured in the study proper. It is usually just one (sometimes lengthy) paragraph. It captures the essence of the study and is a good starting point for the casual reader. For the serious reader, it provides a good roadmap for the territory ahead.

Introduction. The introduction identifies the purpose of the study, provides an overview of the subject matter, and explains why the research you are about to read is important. For example, if treatment failures for a certain disease are high with currently available therapies, the introduction will explain why a more dependable therapy is needed. The introduction usually brings you up to date on recent research regarding the subject matter.

Methods. An explanation of methods provides the credibility that allows the reader to conclude, "Yes, this study is objective and the statistical methods are valid," or, perhaps, "This study design is weak and did not include a large enough sample of patients, nor did the subject include elderly patients (or black patients, or patients with cardiovascular disease)."

I won't get into study protocols, design models, and statistical analysis here. You will learn about these issues during your training. As technical and complex as these issues may be, it is absolutely critical that you understand them. Physicians whom you call on will expect you to have a high level of knowledge about clinical research and to understand such matters as the distinctions to be made among single-blind, double-blind, placebo-controlled, dose-ranging, parallel, and crossover studies.

Results. This is where the study gets *really* technical. The results detail—and I do mean detail—the effects of the treatments under study. The results section often features several pages of dry, purely statistical evidence, accompanied by complex charts, tables, and graphs. If you are discussing a study during a sales call, the physician will be particularly interested in data about your product that is "statistically significant" (see box).

Discussion. Sometimes called "Conclusions," this section of the study includes the interpretations of the researchers. The language in this section is usually more reader-friendly, and examination of this section will tell you whether or not the researchers considered treatment with a certain medication to be successful.

The discussion always reconnects the reader to the purpose of the study. Thus, if the purpose of the study was to determine the efficacy of a 40 mg dose of a certain antibiotic in children under age 12 with otitis media (ear infection), then the discussion, in so many words, will state that the drug either was or was not effective.

References. The references section lists other clinical studies and journal articles the researchers consulted relating to the study. It's not uncommon for a study to have fifty or more endnotes referring to prior research on the subject at hand.

Statistical Significance

In a clinical study, statistical significance is otherwise known as the "confidence level" or "P value." If study results show a statistical significance of .05 (or P =.05), this means that the there was only a 5% chance that the results were due to chance. P=.01 means that there was only a 1% chance the results were due to chance.

Conversely, you could state that the analysis suggested results (e.g., the disease was eradicated) were 95% (or 99%) due to the treatment.

Obviously, the lower the P value, the less likely it is that results are due to chance.

It's important to note that not all clinical studies that you use will specifically relate to the usefulness of your product. Many studies—a far greater number, actually—will be more general in nature. The SLEEPO study, for example, did not evaluate the efficacy and safety of a particular therapy. Instead, it claimed that the correction of anemia with erythropoietin therapy (platelet-replacement drugs) had a beneficial effect regarding sleep disorders among dialysis patients.

It follows that, if your company markets a beneficial platelet replacement drug, then one can safely conclude that it would help alleviate sleeping disorders in dialysis patients. Maybe this would be a big selling point for such a product. In other words, you may often use a study to set up the context in which you will promote your product.

When using a reprint, always mention the following points:
- The principal investigator's name (first name listed on the article).
- The journal's name and publication date.
- The purpose and design of the study.
- The results of study.

- How the results relate to a key product benefit (very important). Examples of benefit statements might be:
- *What this means to you, doctor is*...you will have the confidence that your patients will get the 24-hour blood pressure control they need.
- *What this means to your patients is*...they can continue their daily routines without being slowed down with frustrating side effects.
- *What this means for the health plan is*...patients are less likely to require additional office visits, thus the plan saves money.

The following table provides you with some dos and don'ts regarding the use of clinical papers during sales calls:

Sales Tips for Clinical Reprints

Do	Don't
• *Focus on key points.* Stress items that support the unique advantages of your product.	• *Fumble around for the doctor's copy.* have the reprint ready *before* the call, or know precisely where to locate it.
• *Hand the doctor a clean copy after your presentation.* Do not use your "demo" copy or a copy that is dog-eared, marked up, or highlighted.	• *Read the reprint.* Instead, recite key points from memory.
• *Integrate sales aid.* Use the reprint to support key selling messages.	• *Hand the reprint to the doctor during your presentation.* This takes attention away from your verbal presentation. Present the doctor's copy when you are through speaking.
• *Make eye contact with the doctor.* Remember, you are engaged in conversation with your customer.	• *Point to text passages.* Stick with headlines and tables, which are easier to see.
• *Use pen as pointer.* And point only to clearly identifiable headlines and tables. Your objective is to help the doctor recall the location of key information.	• *Leave a highlighted or marked-up reprint.* The FDA forbids this. Doctors know how to skim reprints. They will find the key points without your help.
• *Translate technical information into tangible benefit.* You are selling a product. Tie the data into a selling message, parallel to what's presented in the sales aid.	• *Use more than one reprint during the sales call.* You will be fortunate to have the doctor read and remember just one reprint. Save the others for future calls.
• *Plan ahead.* Be familiar with the content, and mentally rehearse the use of the reprint before you enter the office.	• *Leave a reprint without making selling point.* Always connect the study's conclusion to a key product benefit.
• *Note physician's association with author.* If the physician has studied with the author, attended lectures, etc., make note of this connection during your presentation.	
• *Plan for follow-up.* Present the paper, ask the physician to read it when he/she has time, and request a follow-up visit.	

Product sampling

Product sampling is one of the most widely used strategies in pharmaceutical marketing.

As mentioned earlier, most (not all) companies provide their representatives with ample supplies of samples. A key part of your day-to-day selling activity requires you to leave samples with the physicians (strictly following FDA sampling practices), and monitoring physician use of the samples.

Yes, samples are "freebies," but they deliver some very tangible benefits to everyone involved—physicians, nurses, health plans, patients, your company, and you.

Here's how:

- Samples allow doctors and nurses a chance to see, touch, and read about the product (from the PI) anytime that's convenient to them.
- Samples provide doctors and nurses with opportunities to see a product "in action" regarding its efficacy, safety, convenience, and patients' likes and dislikes.
- Free samples save money for health plans and patients. Very often, in cases of acute illnesses or infections, samples provide the cure and no one spends any money. If a product doesn't work or is not well tolerated by patients, no transactions occur at the prescription counter and the physician can move on to another therapy.
- Patients enjoy receiving samples from physicians. Samples are tangible (vs. the paper prescription) items, represent a sign of goodwill, and people enjoy receiving "free" merchandise.
- Samples benefit your company by providing exposure for your products, especially new products or products with new dosing strengths or delivery methods.
- Samples benefit you because they provide you with solid reasons for visiting physician offices, either to deliver samples, to check on stocks, or to discuss results with physicians.

Sampling strategies and tactics

"Working the sample closet" is a critical strategy for every sales representative. (A "sample closet" can actually be an entire room, a closet, or a large cabinet.) Some physician practices won't let representatives go near the sample closets. Other practices may allow you to inspect the closet shelves, but only with permission and when accompanied by a physician or nurse. At a few practices, where you are trusted, you are more or less free to roam and inspect the shelves on your own.

When possible, you should always keep a close eye on your company's samples and competitors' samples to determine rates at which they are moving off the shelves. As a rule of thumb, most representatives will visit each physician's office every three or four weeks and leave approximately the same quantity of samples on each visit, unless physicians make special requests. Quantities depend on the size of the practice: more for large group practices, fewer for small practices.

Standard procedure is for the physician to provide a three- or four-day supply of free drug (or a two- to three-week supply for chronic conditions), then write a prescription for the patient to fill if there are no side effects. The physician will usually follow up by phone with the patient ensure that all is going well.

Here was my pet peeve regarding sampling:

On countless occasions, I would be leaving or entering a physician's office and notice a patient leaving the office with enough free samples of my product to stem an epidemic. This usually happens because the patient was particularly pushy for samples, or more likely, the doctor or the nurse is "supplementing" the patient.

When this occurrence is suspected, you need to address the issue with the physician in a tactful manner—immediately. Advise the physician that you observed the patient with all the samples and that your company's sample quantities are limited. Suggest to the physician that other patients, especially patients who are new to the office or newly diagnosed, may represent better candidates for the samples.

If patients do not have insurance coverage and cannot pay for medications on their own, most companies offer indigent patient programs in these situations, and it is usually very easy for physicians to enroll patients in these programs. When appropriate, remind physicians of your company's programs for indigent patients.

Watch for opportunities to make sales presentations to physicians in or near the sample closet. It's a matter of being in the right place at the right time. If you are in the closet and a physician approaches to select some samples, you have an opportunity to sell. This is where the 30-second sales call (covered in the previous chapter) comes into play. On some days at busy group practices, you can deliver three or four presentations just by hanging out near the closet. Just don't loiter—have a reason for being there.

Many rooms or closets are a complete mess. This happens because representatives are constantly rearranging products to make certain their products are positioned more prominently than those of the competition. It may be okay for you to do some housecleaning, but always request permission to do so.

You'll note that packaging for samples is absurdly oversized when you consider that only a few tablets or capsules are inside. This is because pharmaceutical companies apply the same concept to sample displays as retail marketers do; the bigger the packaging and the bolder the colors, the more likely you are to attract customers' attention.

Some physicians and nurses complain about sample packaging. They will tell you that it takes up too much space. Let them know that you understand their concerns, and promise to let your company know how the customer feels (and be sure to follow up by communicating through appropriate internal channels). In the meantime, don't be alarmed if, between sales calls, the customer removes the product from the packaging in order to save space. Don't worry about this. Your responsibility is to provide the product in its original packaging, complete with the package insert.

Snow job

I once drove up to a physician's office in the middle of a heavy snow-storm. The doctor was outside shoveling. He told me that he really needed samples of the product but did not have time for a conversation because he needed to get the driveway cleared before his patients arrived.

I replied to him that I would be happy to leave samples and that my district manager—who happened to be with me that day—would shovel while we spoke. My DM looked at me and grimaced (as if to say "You're gonna buy me a big lunch for this one") and started shoveling. What an effective method for getting some face time with a busy physician!

It is very effective to use samples as part of an "action close." When you ask for a commitment to prescribe the product, present samples of the product to keep on his or her desk for the next patient with the appropriate affliction.

Frequent prescribers of your products should get extra sample attention. Consider visiting them every two weeks and perhaps leaving an extra carton or two.

It's critically important to reload your detail bag with samples after *every* call. You should anticipate how many samples you will need for the day and stock your car. You don't want to run out when you are two hours away from your storage unit.

My final words on sampling are: (1) Use discretion. Don't oversample. Your objective, after all, is to generate paid prescriptions. (2) Follow up with physicians to determine success rates and patient responses—and to ask for prescription business.

Chapter 10

The Managed Care Marketplace

In Chapter 4, I emphasized how important it is for pharmaceutical sales representatives to become familiar with managed care. I cautioned that it is not enough simply to know a product's features and benefits. I also stressed that you need to understand key managed care and business issues confronting physicians in your territory. Without this knowledge, you will be at a severe competitive disadvantage.

Fortunately, most companies provide new representatives with some level of managed care training—anything from handing out a manual and saying "Read this book," to delivering extensive two- or three-day workshops at which your performance will be measured.

Because managed care dominates healthcare in so many parts of the country and influences the ways in which physicians will make decisions regarding your products, I'm including a brief Q&A chapter on managed care basics, with emphasis on managed care's relationship with pharmaceuticals.

What is managed care?

Managed care is a method for organizing healthcare providers (physicians, hospitals, pharmacies, etc.) in an attempt to control healthcare costs and manage the quality of care. In most cases, care is "managed" through a centralized, structured organization such as a health maintenance organization (HMO), preferred provider organization (PPO), or integrated healthcare system.

Managed care is now the dominant form of healthcare delivery in the United States because of public and private frustration with skyrocketing healthcare costs among:

- employers (who pay for healthcare premiums)
- the government (which pays for Medicare and Medicaid)
- consumers (who, in the end, pay for it all)

These constituencies told providers "Enough!" and turned to managed care organizations (MCOs) to clamp the lid on healthcare costs.

Does managed care work?

Although managed care has not eliminated the problem of constantly escalating healthcare costs, it has, for the most part, helped to keep annual increases at tolerable levels by:

- managing the use of healthcare services (largely by controlling patient access to specialized care and eliminating unnecessary and redundant services)
- limiting provider fees (by establishing capitated rates for physician and hospital services)
- controlling drug costs (by implementing managed pharmacy benefit programs, formularies, copayment arrangements, and other cost-control tools)

How does managed care differ from traditional indemnity insurance?

Managed care differs from traditional indemnity insurance plans. In these plans patients (usually through their employers) pay premiums to cover the cost of care. In that system providers get paid by submitting claims to insurers *after* a service is provided.

In managed care, providers are paid *before* providing any services. By paying providers prospectively, MCOs (which are really insurance companies) force *providers* to assume financial risk for the services they provide.

The most common prospective payment system is called "capitation." A capitated payment is a prepayment for services by a health plan to a provider on a per member per month (pmpm) basis.

Thus, if a certain physician group practice contracts with an MCO to provide services for 200 members for a pmpm fee of $150, the MCO pays the group $30,000 each month (200 x $150) regardless of the extent to which the members require care—*even if they require no care at all.*

What role do pharmaceuticals play in managed care?

Pharmaceuticals play a vital role in managed care. Prescription drugs can help MCOs achieve their goals by:
- accelerating the recovery of patients with short-term illness
- simplifying management of chronically ill patients
- providing lower-cost alternatives to other treatment methods (e.g., surgery)

Because managed care focuses heavily on cost controls, providers must try to provide *cost-effective* pharmaceutical care. Thus, it's important that sales representatives remain aware of how managed care is sensitive to the cost of your products.

How do MCOs try to control prescription drug costs?

MCOs use a number of strategies to control drug costs, and you need to be familiar with all that apply to your products.

Virtually all MCOs try to manage prescription drug costs by implementing a pharmacy benefit program. Essentially, a pharmacy benefit program includes prescription drugs as part of healthcare coverage, either incorporated into the basic premium or, sometimes, for an optional separate premium. If part of a patient's care includes prescription drugs, the plan pays for all or part of the prescription cost.

Usually, patients covered by a pharmacy benefit must fill their prescriptions at specified retail pharmacies that participate in a health plan's retail pharmacy network. These pharmacies provide drugs at discounts (usually paid in the form of volume-based rebates) to MCOs in exchange for guaranteed patient volume.

Typically, when filling prescriptions at these pharmacies, plan members must provide the retail pharmacist with an out-of-pocket copayment.

What's a copayment?

Copayments are fixed fees (e.g., $5 or $10) that help shift the cost of prescription drugs from the plan to the consumer. The objective of copayments is to help discourage unnecessary drug use.

Many plans use tiered copayments to promote the use of less expensive generic products or preferred branded products (which usually cost less than nonpreferred brands). Under a tiered copayment system, a patient might, for example, provide a copayment of $5 for a generic drug, $10 for a preferred brand, and $15 for a nonpreferred brand.

What's a formulary?

A managed care formulary is a list of plan-approved drugs designed to encourage physicians to prescribe the most cost-effective medications.

Most MCOs use drug formularies to help reduce the cost of prescription drugs.

Formularies typically include lower-priced generic products and may exclude higher-priced branded products. Plans request or require physicians to use formulary drugs unless there is a valid medical reason to use another product.

Formulary enforcement varies. Some formularies are "open" and allow physicians to prescribe almost any product, although certain restrictions may apply. A high copayment for a nonpreferred brand or a nonformulary product is an example of a restriction.

Another example is a procedure called "prior authorization," which requires the physician to obtain permission from the plan's medical director or chief pharmacist before prescribing a nonpreferred product.

"Closed" formularies are much more restrictive and require physicians to prescribe only from listed drugs.

How are drugs selected for formularies?

A pharmaceutical company must submit a formulary approval request to a health plan's pharmacy and therapeutics (P&T) committee for a drug to be considered. Committees usually consist of the plan's medical director, pharmacy director, a financial specialist, and physicians from key specialties.

P&T committees usually base their formulary decisions on a product's:

- therapeutic appropriateness (Does it meet a clinical need?)
- uniqueness (What makes the product better than its competitors?)
- clinical trial data (Has it been proven to provide clinical advantages?)
- cost (Is it fairly priced? Is it cost-effective, based on anticipated outcomes?)

Normally, a national account manager ushers a product through the formulary approval process. Territory sales representatives may be asked to support the process by providing information to the plan's pharmacy department and to selected physicians. (On many occasions I asked physicians who were committed to my product to write letters of recommendation to P&T committees.)

Formularies are important tools for cost control in managed care, and MCOs expect sales representatives to respect their formularies when promoting products to plan-affiliated physicians. Always make certain that your product is on formulary before promoting it to a physician who is closely linked with a particular MCO.

What is drug utilization review?

Drug utilization review (DUR) refers to an MCO's practice of monitoring prescribing patterns to confirm the appropriateness of drug selections as well as physicians' compliance with a health plan's formulary guidelines and other cost-control procedures.

DUR helps control costs by:
- reducing inappropriate drug use, which may harm patients (e.g., through adverse effects or harmful interactions with other drugs) and increase plan costs
- forcing "errant" physicians (those who fail to follow formulary guidelines) to conform with plan guidelines

Most MCOs use computer reports to review the average number of prescriptions per month (total, by specialty, by individual physician) and the average cost per prescription. Then, analysts compare utilization and costs among individual physicians, groups, or specialties. Plan administrators use the data to evaluate pharmacy costs and to spot opportunities for savings.

If you imagine a bell curve, plans generally consider physicians in the middle zone to be the "norm." Physicians whose prescribing volume falls at either end of the curve (low or high) may receive letters or calls from a medical or pharmacy director to determine the rationale for their abnormal prescribing patterns.

Some plans' computer systems enable pharmacy directors to match drugs to diseases, allowing them to track diseases for which physicians most often prescribe nonformulary drugs and to identify diseases for which physician prescribing patterns are inconsistent.

What's a "PBM"?

A PBM, or "pharmacy benefit manager," is an outside organization hired by a health plan to manage all or part of the plan's pharmacy benefit program. A very high percentage of MCOs and self-insured employers hire PBMs to manage the administrative functions of their pharmacy benefits.

PBMs provide the following services, usually on an a la carte basis:
- claims processing
- formulary management
- drug utilization review
- data processing, management, and reporting
- physician prescribing profiles
- physician education

PBMs also interact with pharmaceutical manufacturers by negotiating volume-discount contracts (through national account managers), managing rebate programs, and providing utilization and market-share data.

PBMs interact with retail pharmacies by adjudicating claims, providing on-line clinical information, and reimbursing retailers (providing a "dispensing fee" from the health plan for every prescription filled for plan members).

From the sales representative's perspective, it's important to know how PBMs fit into the benefit programs offered by local MCOs and large employers in your territory. It is the responsibility of a national account manager or district manager to inform representatives about PBM contracts that affect local selling territories.

What other managed care concepts should a new representative know about?

There are a couple: clinical practice guidelines and disease management.

Clinical practice guidelines. Clinical practice guidelines are systematically developed statements or decision trees ("algorithms" is a frequently used term) that help physicians make informed decisions about appropriate healthcare for specific clinical circumstances.

These guidelines summarize prevailing medical knowledge about a certain disease or condition and recommend specific diagnostic, therapeutic, and medical management protocols.

Guidelines range from simple one-page decision trees to several pages of text (and are often posted on the internet). In effect, clinical practice guidelines are blueprints to help physicians make more informed decisions about treatment options.

Pharmaceuticals play an important role in clinical practice guidelines. When a recommendation for a certain therapeutic category appears in a guideline (guidelines rarely recommend branded products), it shows that the medical community believes that these products provide the desired outcome in specific clinical situations.

If your product's therapeutic category (e.g., an antihypertensive [blood pressure] drug) is mentioned in a practice guideline, then you have a convenient "hook" on which to base a sales presentation.

Disease management. Disease management is a coordinated approach to healthcare that focuses on the entire patient-care continuum for a disease or condition, from prevention of and early screening for that disease, through aftercare and analysis of patient outcomes (i.e., did they get better?).

Disease management can help reduce costs by:

- keeping patients healthy, through preventive healthcare, thus avoiding the need for medical care
- effectively managing (or curing) a disease or condition, thus reducing the demand for additional, expensive services (such as surgery)
- monitoring patient behavior to help ensure that patients manage their lifestyles appropriately and take their prescriptions as directed

Disease management strategies are usually targeted for chronic therapeutic disease categories such as asthma, coronary artery disease (CAD), hypertension, diabetes, cancer, and AIDS. Note that these diseases are expensive to treat and manage, and can be often be effectively managed through pharmaceutical care as an alternative to expensive surgical interventions.

Also—and this is very important from a sales representative's perspective—appropriate pharmaceutical care in the treatment of these diseases can help contribute to improved outcomes while reducing the overall cost of care. For example, appropriate use of inhalation devices by asthma patients can help reduce emergency room visits and expensive inpatient treatment.

Pharmaceutical companies often participate in disease management partnerships with MCOs by providing grant money and support for physician and patient education. The appropriate sales manager will apprise territory sales representatives of disease management programs that influence sales activity in a territory.

What's the role of the territory sales representative in managed care?

At most pharmaceutical companies, national account managers or other senior sales professionals set the stage for field sales representatives by negotiating national contracts at the top of the managed care hierarchy. Contracts established with MCOs (or their PBMs), generally allow MCOs to purchase the drugs at discounts (and/or receive volume-based rebates) in return for placing the products on formulary.

However, even the most comprehensive contracts do not guarantee that physicians will prescribe your products at the territory level. Therefore, the responsibility of the field sales representative is to implement contracts by generating "pull-through" demand among physicians. Without pull-through, a product is merely an entry on a formulary list.

Of course, this involves a lot more than simply showing up and delivering a standard sales presentation to physicians. You must be aware of a product's formulary position, its relative cost, physician financial incentives, disease management programs and clinical practice guidelines, and a lot more.

*   *   *   *   *

A final comment on managed care

Today, the rapid evolution of managed care presents some significant challenges for pharmaceutical sales professionals. You can rarely open a newspaper on any given day without reading about a merger, an acquisition, an MCO expanding into a new market area, Medicare/Medicaid issues in managed care, or a consumer lawsuit against a health plan. Any or all of these issues can influence prescription drug business in a territory.

Thus, no matter how well you understand managed care, you will probably never know enough. Regardless of how well you analyze your territory and position your products today, the scenario will change—tomorrow, next week, or next month. Keeping up with the changes and, more importantly, the impact of those changes on pharmaceutical utilization, is an essential part of the sales representative's job.

Keep in mind that physicians will continue to write the majority of prescriptions for managed care patients, and these physicians *need*

information about your products' clinical advantages, economic benefits, outcomes data, and positioning in MCO practice guidelines and
disease management programs.

Most MCOs recognize that the best source for this information is a
credible pharmaceutical sales representative who *knows* the market,
understands managed care, and *fulfills* the unique needs of all the key
players within the MCO's sphere of influence. These players include
employers, managed care administrators, physicians, pharmacists,
and patients.

If you meet these responsibilities, pull-through success naturally
follows.

Chapter 11

Top 10 Ways to Jump-start Your Pharmaceutical Sales Career

I hope that this book has provided you with an adequate introduction to what a career in pharmaceutical sales is all about. I think you've seen that it is a challenging profession that offers a great deal of intellectual and financial rewards to those who are successful.

If you are thinking about a career in pharmaceutical sales, I hope that my thoughts have provided sufficient encouragement to take the next step. If you have just been hired and are reading this book as part of your orientation, you now have an idea of what lies ahead.

At the end of every training program my colleagues and I always made it a point to briefly present some motivational remarks to participants. My motivational remarks to you are presented in the form of ten techniques that I believe helped me achieve and maintain a high level of success when I was a territory sales representative.

Read and apply them, and you'll have a jump-start on your own successful career in pharmaceutical sales.

1. Display an attitude of gratitude.

Let's face it…Your customers don't need you. You need them.

When a customer does *anything* for you, small or large, never forget to thank that person. Most of the time this means simply saying "thank you" at the right time during a conversation. At other times, it is more appropriate to write a brief thank-you note.

Along the same lines, I always made it a point to purchase and mail holiday cards every year just to thank my customers for their support. These gestures demonstrate your appreciation for their business and keeps your name in front of them in a positive way. It's hard to believe that more representatives do not utilize them more often.

Providing personal attention to your customers in the form of a "thank you" is a powerful method for developing mutually beneficial relationships. Here are a few situations into which it will be easy for you to insert a simple "thank you":

- When a customer responds to your question ("Thanks for the information.")
- After the customer states an objection ("Thank you for expressing your concern.")
- After he or she agrees to sample or prescribe the product ("Thanks for trying Product X.")
- Every time the customer meets with you ("Thanks for your time.")
- When a customer agrees to write or speak on your product's behalf ("Thank you for your support.")
- When a customer shares information about his or her practice ("Thank you for sharing that information with me.")

Be generous in your thanks to receptionists, nurses, and office staff, too.

2. Stay positive, enthusiastic, and confident.

Always remember that your customers deal with sickness and death all day long, day after day. Patients are grumpy, whiny, anxious, and depressed because they simply don't feel well. Patients justifiably feel that way and are expected to behave that way. This makes for a tough job for physicians and their staff. Don't add to it with an indifferent attitude on your part.

Not only do you provide a solution to many of your customer's clinical needs with your products and services, but you have the opportunity to provide a cheerful break in their day. As you'll learn, many of your customers actually *enjoy* your visits. They'll become genuine friends with you and want to hear your humorous stories and discuss sports and hobbies with you.

If you happen to have had a bad experience on a particular day, don't carry it in the customer's office with you. Remember that your customers are "buying" you, too. You want your customers to associate you with good feelings.

Here's a quote about attitude that many sales representatives carry in the field:

> "The longer I live, the more I realize the impact of attitude on life. Attitude, to me, is more important than facts. It is more important than the past, than education, than money, than circumstances, than failures, than successes, than what other people think or say or do. It is more important than appearance, giftedness, or skill. It will make or break a company...a church...a home.
>
> "The remarkable thing is we have a choice every day regarding the attitude we will embrace for that day. We cannot change our past...we cannot change the fact that people will act in a certain way. We cannot change the

inevitable. The only thing we can do is play the one string
we have, and that is our attitude…

"I am certain that life is 10% what happens to me, and
90% how I react to it. And so it is with you…we are in
charge of our attitudes."

—Charles Swindall

3. Be creative. Have fun.

You are hired as a pharmaceutical representative because experienced sales professionals believe that you can not only handle the technical aspects of the job, but also because you bring your own unique style to the job. No one else has your personality and God-given gifts and talents. Always make it a point to have fun and enjoy what you do with this job. Don't be afraid to implement interesting ideas, strategies, and tactics that you and your customers will both enjoy. (Just make sure you stay within FDA regulations regarding drug promotions.)

I always had a lot of fun playing with words and phrases. Sometimes the customers would say things such as "Did they actually teach you to say that?" in response to a tongue-in-cheek play on words or a really bad pun. That was a great response to me.

If there are methods you can employ to improve your customer's office efficiency or expand his or her practice by all means do it. A former supervisor of mine loved to use the example of a representative who organized computer skills training for a physician's office staff when they were having a hard time with a new system. After that gesture, he virtually owned the office!

I know of another representative who loved baseball and played it in college before launching his sales career. One of the most successful medical education programs he organized involved physicians attending a captivating clinical presentation inside a lecture hall while he provided batting instruction for their children on an adjacent playing field.

Some sales gurus have told me that imagination is more important than intellect. I think there is a degree of truth in this. You will rarely, if ever, achieve the higher level of clinical knowledge that a physician customer possesses. However, when you combine your relatively inferior knowledge with a little imagination, there are few limits to what you can achieve in a sales setting.

As a trainer I enjoyed role playing with a representative who used his knowledge of magic to open and close his presentations—I really looked forward to his role plays because of that. He used the same techniques in the field.

In fact, when it comes to your imagination in this business, the sky is the limit! One of my most successful programs was a medical education speaker program that I scheduled at the city science museum. After the lecture and dinner, the physicians (particularly the residents) behaved like young children while watching a laser show in the planetarium.

4. Love your family. Like your job.

Your job will take you away to meetings and workshops for days at a time. You will host many programs in the evenings. There will be times during the weekend when you must wrap up the previous week or prepare for the upcoming week.

Despite all of these responsibilities, you must make sure to schedule quality time with your significant other, your family, and friends. You must devote at least the same amount of energy and enthusiasm to meeting your family's needs as you do with your customers. Many new representatives have lofty career ambitions for money, promotions, sales success, and recognition. That's fine—just don't let such an attitude rule your life. Maintain an appropriate balance, and prioritize what is most important to you.

5. Nurture your customer relationships.

Always make it a point to be customer-friendly. Be easy to get in touch with. Be approachable and genuinely open to conversation. Ask questions about your customer's hobbies, interests, hopes, and dreams. Share yours as well. Always smile and call people by their names. If you're like most of us and forget names easily, make it a point to write them down.

Many nonphysicians in the healthcare community play very important supportive roles in pharmaceutical decision-making—pharmacists, nurses, lab technicians, office administrators, physician assistants, nurse practitioners, and so on. It is essential that you make them feel important for what they do. Always take time to speak with them. You never know when they might be able to provide you with a favor or two.

Here are some "nurturing" tips that I practiced over the years:

- Provide information to the staff on a regular basis. Keep them informed about new products at your company.
- Ask if you can see "their" physician.
- Say "Doctor, that is a great point. Many physicians I see feel the same way."
- Get to know the entire office staff, and include everyone in luncheons.
- Say something positive to everyone you meet.

6. Hold yourself accountable.

As a mature adult, you alone are responsible for your successes and failures. Troubled past experiences and tough current circumstances simply represent steppingstones for greater achievement.

Don't forget that one of the reasons why you were hired is to solve problems (sometimes big ones) for your company and your customers—now, *that's* opportunity.

You have probably observed—or even experienced—in life how easy it is for people to blame others for their own shortcomings. In my career, I heard such excuses as "the marketing department did not provide good studies," or "the training department was not realistic."

Learn to recognize when you—and others—are simply making excuses. As a professional, you must be acutely aware of your own strengths and weaknesses. Determine what steps you need to take to improve your sales, your career, and your situation. Take action and implement steps with an eye on crafting the future as you see it. Visualization is a powerful tool. Create your vision, then take steps to make it come true.

Also, maintaining your integrity and character is critical in sales. If you don't have the answer, tell them and then follow up with the answer. Sell within the rules of the FDA, managed care organizations, physician offices, and your company.

It's often tempting to bend the rules when no one is looking. I know of representatives who "sneak" into sample closets to rearrange products when staff members are not around. Forget about it. Don't risk losing a customer. Do the *right* thing when no one is looking.

7. Practice self-discipline.

There will be many times when you won't want to put in the necessary time to study a learning module or prepare a sales report for your manager. Regardless of the circumstances, you must make it a habit to accomplish the tasks that you don't like to do. It's very much like the long-distance runner who gets out of a warm and comfortable bed every morning to train in the cold for the upcoming race. It takes discipline and persistence.

It's not a matter of avoiding those behaviors that inevitably lead to failure (such as working only until 3 p.m. everyday or not planning for sales calls). It is a matter of *proactively* doing the right things. For example, you must set regular goals and objectives, then create tactics that will allow you to achieve your dreams. Do you want to be in the

President's Club for outstanding sales achievement? Do you want to go on the all-expense paid vacation to the islands? If the answers are "yes," write down the goals and write down the steps you need to complete in order to accomplish those goals.

Here are some other activities that will help you fine-tune your self-discipline:

- Read and re-read appropriate journal articles on a regular basis.
- Monitor curricula offered by your company and local universities. Take appropriate courses on a regular basis. (Your company may reimburse you for tuition.)
- Be consistent every day with your sales methods and messages. Sometimes it will take months for you to change a physician's prescribing habits.
- Visualize sales success. Focus in your mind each day completing each step along the way to reaching your ultimate goal.
- Practice fundamental selling skills every day. You never know when the game is on the line. Larry Bird won many basketball games with free throws, which he practiced for hours in an empty gym. He rarely missed because he knew that practicing the fundamentals is essential to success.
- Maintain your credibility and professionalism with your customers by always staying on top of your game and being politely persistent.

8. Spend most of your time with your most important customers.

The 80/20 rule is alive and well. Eighty percent of your business will come from 20% of your customers. Take note of where your business is coming from, and take the time each quarter for proper territory and account planning. Investment up front with all those company reports will pay off with high prescription volume for you in the end.

Keep an eye on the future, too. Constantly scout your territory to determine the source of future high-prescribers. Perhaps it is a new group practice in an important zip code or a new doctor on staff at a busy practice. Spend time cultivating these prospects, and you'll be rewarded with valuable long-term relationships and higher numbers at the end of every quarter.

9. Listen to your customer.

I talked about listening skills in Chapter 7. Most of the time, the information you need in order to gain a physician's commitment to prescribe your product will not be readily available to you. You must ask well chosen open-ended questions and encourage the customer to continue and expand what they are saying. Be sincerely interested in the response.

Joe Sinopoli, a high-level pharmacy administrator at Harvard Pilgrim Health Care in Boston once said, "Don't tell me what you think I want to hear. Tell me what I need to know." And the only way you will find out what Joe or anyone else needs to know is to listen carefully to what they say. Sinopoli says that, time after time, he extrapolates at length (Joe is a big talker) to representatives on what his department's needs are. Yet, he says, few representatives really listen. "All they want to do is give their canned presentations," he says.

Don't be one of these representatives. The point is that despite all your selling skills and clinical knowledge you really must let the *customer* control the call. When you think about it, it makes perfect sense. You need to learn what motivates your customers, to anticipate what their key concerns and objections might be, and to identify their expectations (and their patients' expectations) regarding you, your company, and your products.

And don't forget, you set yourself up to be a good listener by asking good questions.

10. Be proud of what you do

You'll hear all the time—in the media, from friends and relatives, and the proverbial "man on the street"—about the "greed" and "profit-mongering" of big pharmaceutical companies.

Don't let it wear you down. You're in a great industry and it's a great time to be in that industry. Be confident that you represent a critically important solution in today's healthcare marketplace. You bring value to customers because you educate and inform them about products and support programs that not only help people get better, but save money, too, in terms of reducing demand on expensive services, such as surgery and hospital stays.

In the final analysis, you are the critical link between the problem (patients who want to improve their health) and the solution (safe, effective medications).

It is not a reach to conclude that the pharmaceutical industry helps to enhance and extend the lives of millions of people every day, and that you are the face of that industry in the eyes of the half-million doctors across the country.

Have a great career!

About the Authors

David Currier is currently a performance improvement manager for a premier biotechnology company. Previously, he was a consultant to the pharmaceutical industry at a training firm. He also worked at a leading pharmaceutical corporation for several years as a sales representative and sales training manager.

Jay Frost is a freelance writer who has authored several books on managed care. He has also prepared the text for dozens of pharmaceutical sales training manuals, newsletters, workshops, audio/visual scripts, CD ROM programs, and websites.

Appendix

Other Books on Pharmaceutical Sales Careers

The Art of Pharmaceutical Selling: A Professional Medical Representative's Guide to Successful Selling Skills, Stockton, CA: Coastec Inc., 1997 (207-476-0670). A wide-ranging handbook that covers key selling skills. Topics include profiling customers, precall planning, selling tools, listening and questioning, objection-handling, relations with retail pharmacies, and more.

Bischoff, Martin B., *Successful Pharmaceutical Selling,* New York: McGraw-Hill, 1997. ISBN 0-7863-1211-4. A basic guide for day-to-day selling techniques, with special attention to both physicians and hospitals, two vastly different markets. Covers teamwork, competitive issues, ethics, sales resources, managed care, and more.

Clayton, Anne, *Insight into a Career in Pharmaceutical Sales* (2nd edition), Northbrook, IL: Marketing Essentials Incorporated, 1999. (*www.pharmaceutical-sales.com*). ISBN 0-9665 121-1-1. A comprehensive guide to landing your first sales job in pharmaceuticals. Includes industry background information, job search and interview tips, cover letters, interview guidelines, company profiles, and worksheets.

Internet Resources

Medical Sales Associates
Jobs for sales and marketing professionals in the pharmaceutical and biotech industries.
http://www.msajobs.com

Pharmaceutical Sales Representative
Free advice, tips and information on how to land a job as a pharmaceutical sales representative from the perspective of a field sales veteran.
http://www.coreynahman.com/practicaladvice.html

Pharmaceutical, Medical Sales
Advice for job candidates. Specializing in oncology, infectious diseases and biotech sales.
http://home.att.net/~dyh15

Insider's Guide to the World of Pharmaceutical Sales
A job-seeker's guide on how to secure a job in Pharmaceutical Sales.
http://www.principlepublications.com

Pharmaceutical Sales Employment Guide
Information about sales careers in the pharmaceutical industry.
http://pages.preferred.com/~slade

Pharmaceutical Sales Positions

Tips for landing a career in pharmaceutical sales. Suggestions for resume development and interview preparation.

http://mo-info.com

Pharmaceutical Training

Advice and resources for sales training managers, sales personnel, and job seekers.

http://www.pharmtraining.com

Major U.S. Pharmaceutical Companies

Visit company websites for information about products and employment opportunities. For summary descriptions of each company, see Appendix A in **Insight into a Career in Pharmaceutical Sales,** *by Anne Clayton, available from Marketing Essentials Incorporated, 835 Sanders Road, #167, Northbrook, IL, 60062 (www.pharmaceutical-sales.com).*

Abbott Laboratories
100 Abbott Park Road
Abbott Park, IL 60064
(847) 937-6100
http://www.abbott.com
http://www.Rxabbott.com

Akzo Nobel NV
Organon Incorporated
375 Mount Pleasant Avenue
West Orange, NJ 07052
(973) 325-4589
http://akznobel.com

American Home Products Corporation
Wyeth Laboratories
5 Giralda Farms
Madison, NJ 07940
(201) 660-5000
http://www.ahp.com

Amgen Incorporated
1840 DeHavilland Drive
Thousand Oaks, CA 91320
(805) 447-1000
http://www.amgen.com

Astra Zeneca
50 Otis Street
Westborough, MA 01581
(508) 366-1100
http://www.astra.com

Aventis
(Rhone Poulenc Rorer/Hoechst Marion Merrell Dow)
PO Box 9627
Kansas City, MO 64134
(816) 966-5000
http://www.hmri.com

BASF
Knoll Pharmaceutical Company
3000 Continental Drive–North
Mount Olive, NJ 07828
(973) 426-6000
http://www.basf.de

Bausch & Lomb
One Bausch & Lomb Place
Rochester, NY 14604
(716) 338-6000
http://www.bausch.com

Bayer Corporation
500 Grant Street
Pittsburgh, PA
(412) 394-5500
http://www.bayer-ag.de

Boehringer-Ingelheim Corporation
900 Ridgebury Road
Ridgefield, CT 06877
http://www.boehringer-ingelheim.com

Bristol-Myers Squibb Company
345 Park Avenue
New York, NY 10154
(212) 546-4000
http://www.bms.com

E.I. Du Pont de Nemours and Co.
974 Centre Road
Wilmington, DE 19898
(302) 774-1000
http://www.dupontpharma.com

Eli Lilly and Company
Lilly Corporate Center
Indianapolis, IN 46285
(317) 276-2000
http://www.lilly.com

Genentech
1 DBA Way
South San Francisco, CA 94080
(650) 225-1000
http://www.gene.com

Glaxo-Wellcome PLC
Five Moore Drive
Research Triangle Park, NC 27709
(919)-483-0084
http://www.glaxowellcome.co.uk
Johnson and Johnson
One Johnson and Johnson Plaza
New Brunswick, NJ, 08993
(732) 524-0400
http://www.jnj.com

Merck and Company Inc.
One Merck Drive
Whitehouse Station, NJ 08889
(908) 423-1000
http://www.merck.com

3M (Minnesota Mining and Manufacturing Company)
3M Center
St. Paul, MN 55144
(651) 733-1110
http://www.mmm.com

Monsanto (G.D. Searle Incorporated)
800 North Lindbergh Boulevard
St. Louis, MO 63167
(314) 694-1000
http://www.monsanto.com

Novartis
556 Morris Avenue
Summit, NJ 07901
(908) 277-5293
http://www.novartis.com

Novo Nordisk A/S
405 Lexington Avenue, Suite 6400
New York, NY 10017
(212) 867-0123
http://www.novo.dk

Pfizer Incorporated
235 East 42nd Street
New York, NY 10017
(212) 573-2323
http://www.pfizer.com

Pharmacia & Upjohn Inc.
7000 Portage Road
Kalamazoo, MI 49001
(616) 833-4000
http://www.pharmacia.se

Procter & Gamble
One Procter & Gamble Plaza
Cincinnati, OH 45202
(513) 983-1100
http://www.pg.com

Roberts Pharmaceutical Corporation
Meridian Center II
4 Industrial Way West
Eatontown, NJ 07724
(732) 389-1182
http://www.robertspharm.com

Roche Holding AG
340 Kingsland Street
Nutley, NJ 07110
(973) 235-5000
http://www.roche.com

Sanofi-Synthelabo Pharmaceuticals
90 Park Avenue
New York, NY 10016
(212) 907-3368
http://www.sanofi-winthrop.com

Schering-Plough Corporation
One Giralda Farms
Madison, NJ 07940
(973) 822-7000
http://www.schering-plough.com

Serono
100 Longwater Circle
Norwell, MA 02061
http://www.seronousa.com

SmithKline Beecham PLC
1 Franklin Plaza
PO Box 7929
Philadelphia, PA 19101
(215) 751-5166
http://www.sb.com

Solvay
901 Sawyer Road
Marietta, GA 30062
(770) 578-9000
http://www.solvay.com

Warner-Lambert Company
Parke-Davis
201 Tabor Road
Morris Plains, NJ 07950
(973) 540-2000
http://www.warner-lambert.com

0-595-17418-3